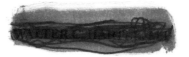

PRACTICAL TECHNIQUES IN
OPHTHALMIC
PLASTIC SURGERY

PRACTICAL TECHNIQUES IN
OPHTHALMIC
PLASTIC SURGERY

BYRON C. SMITH, M.D.

Clinical Professor of Ophthalmology, Senior Consultant to
the Ophthalmic Plastic Service, Manhattan Eye,
Ear and Throat Hospital, New York, New York

FRANK A. NESI, M.D.

Chief of Eye Plastic Service, Kresge Eye Institute;
Clinical Instructor, Department of Ophthalmology,
Wayne State University School of Medicine, Detroit, Michigan

with **307** illustrations in **69** plates
by **Virginia Hoyt Cantarella, A.M.I.**

The C. V. Mosby Company

ST. LOUIS • TORONTO • LONDON   1981

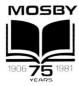

A TRADITION OF PUBLISHING EXCELLENCE

Editor: Eugenia A. Klein
Assistant editor: Kathryn H. Falk
Manuscript editor: Sally Gaines
Design: Jeanne Bush
Production: Debbie Wedemeier

Printed in the United States of America

The C.V. Mosby Company
11830 Westline Industrial Drive, St. Louis, Missouri 63141

Library of Congress Cataloging in Publication Data

Smith, Byron, 1908-
  Practical techniques in ophthalmic plastic
surgery.

  Bibliography: p.
  Includes index.
  1. Adnexa oculi—Surgery. 2. Surgery, Plastic.
I. Nesi, Frank A., 1944-   . II. Title. [DNLM:
1. Eye—Surgery—Atlases. 2. Surgery, Plastic—
Atlases. WW 17 S643p]
RE87.S66   617.7'1   81-11105
ISBN 0-8016-4662-6   AACR2

TS/CB/B   9 8 7 6 5 4 3 2 1   03/C/309

PREFACE

The preparation of this book was stimulated by our desire to update the technical details of a limited number of surgical procedures that we use frequently. Most of the operative methods were originated by others. The simple drawings and descriptive, concise text provide the details of the surgical approach to a number of frequently encountered abnormalities. The details and modifications are depicted and described in accordance with the methods we currently use.

We admit that it is much easier to draw diagrams of our operations than it is to perform the same procedure on living tissue. As in any other artistic endeavor, the results are dependent on the skill and artistic ability of the surgeon. It is beyond the scope of this book to alter these attributes in any individual surgeon. The suggestions contained in this publication are meant to crystallize the technical details and minimize the possibilities of complication and failure.

We are grateful to all those responsible for the original contributions to the field of ophthalmic plastic surgery. Had it not been for their originality and generosity, it would have been impossible to compile the contents of this book. In addition, we are grateful to all those responsible for our training and to those responsible for stimulating us to contribute additional knowledge to the field. Daisy Stilwell shall always be remembered for her many fine drawings that have proven helpful to Virginia Cantarella in the finalization of her artistic accomplishments in this book. We wish to thank Virginia Cantarella for her artistic ability and her many helpful suggestions. Our appreciation is also expressed to Dr. Garron Klepack for his suggestions in the sections on preoperative evaluation. Finally, we appreciate the efforts of those hospitals, clinics, referring physicians, nurses, technicians, and all others responsible for our accomplishments.

Byron C. Smith
Frank A. Nesi

CONTENTS

PRACTICAL TECHNIQUES IN
OPHTHALMIC
PLASTIC SURGERY

CHAPTER 1

EVALUATION OF THE PATIENT

The preoperative evaluation of the patient about to undergo ophthalmic plastic or reconstructive surgery should begin with a consideration of the patient's attitude toward and expectations about surgery. The surgeon should give a candid appraisal of the anticipated results of surgery and should speak with sensitivity about that which is certainly an important matter for the patient—his personal appearance. This is of primary importance in establishing a good relationship with the patient and avoiding future difficulties. It is essential that the patient's expectations of the surgical results approximate reasonably achievable goals for the surgeon.

Preoperative photographic documentation of the patient is an integral part of the initial examination. We use a Kodak Instamatic camera in the office and routinely order 35 mm color slides and 5 × 7 black and white photographs to be taken at the time of hospital admission.

A complete ophthalmic examination should be performed on every patient regardless of the type of case. A corrected visual acuity is obtained. If indicated, visual field testing is performed by tangent screen or Goldman-type perimetry. In an unresponsive patient, examination of the pupils may indicate an afferent pupillary defect and therefore a monocular optic nerve lesion. (In a traumatic case, a paralysis of the iris or iris sphincter may result from a traumatic rupture.) An efferent pupillary defect is signified by a poor response to light directly or consensually and may indicate a compressive or traumatic lesion of the third nerve.

An external examination will reveal asymmetries of contour that may be within normal limits, as well as eyelid malpositions, lack of lid tonicity, cutaneous defects (scarring), and globe malposition (enophthalmus and exophthalmus). These abnormalities should be pointed out to the patient preoperatively. Baseline exophthalmometry measurements should be performed when indicated.

Slit lamp examination of the conjunctiva can reveal cicatricial inflammation and injury from chemical or thermal burns, Stevens-Johnson syndome, pemphigoid, or an infectious process. As sequelae of these, scarring and deformity of the lids with entropion and trichiasis may result. The lacrimal ducts may be ablated, producing a dry eye. Small tumors of the lids and periorbita should be noted and suspicious lesions excised with clean surgical margins. The medial canthi should be carefully examined because of the dire consequences of late excision in this area.

A motility examination done at near and far in the cardinal fields of gaze is useful, because extraocular muscle imbalance is often associated with congenital defects, traumatic injury, or orbital tumors.

Quantification done preoperatively not only may reveal the extent of ocular involvement but also may provide a baseline for postoperative evaluation.

Direct and indirect opthalmoscopy following dilatation is also useful in revealing congenital defects and traumatic injury. Fundus abnormalities must be noted and documented preoperatively, because they may have a bearing on postoperative results.

The lacrimal system should be evaluated by the performance of secretory and excretory tests. A Schirmer No. 1 test to measure reflex and basic secretion should be performed first. Following the instillation of anesthetic solution, the basic secretors should be tested alone. Primary and secondary dye tests should then be performed to test the excretory mechanism. This testing is essential not only in cases of epiphora but also as a baseline in ptosis and blepharoplasty surgery in which a slight overcorrection may cause a dry eye syndrome.

The ophthalmologist performing plastic or reconstructive surgery should use the expertise of related specialists. For example, personally reviewing the radiographs with the radiologist enhances the clinical information from the variety of techniques available. While plain films of the facial bones and skull may reveal the obvious fracture or foreign body, polytomography in coronal, submental vertex, or sagittal planes can document what are otherwise merely clinical suspicions. High resolution computerized tomography (CT scan) in axial, coronal, and third-dimensional projections are evaluated. Density measurement techniques of the CT scan, particularly when combined with orbital A-scan ultrasound, provide considerable information on the nature and pathology of the lesion. The apex is no longer the safe harbor of orbital pathology. Tumors and vascular abnormalities of the orbit or cranium presenting with orbital signs require cerebral angiography of the external and internal circulation to document full anatomic features of the feeding and draining blood supply. The proper course of therapy may include the assistance of the neurologist, neurosurgeon, otolaryngologist, or maxillofacial surgeon in a cooperative surgical effort.

CHAPTER 2

ANATOMIC CORRELATION

To successfully perform plastic or reconstructive surgery of the ocular adnexa, one needs a thorough knowledge of orbital and eyelid anatomy. The success of split-thickness skin or composite dermis-fat grafting techniques depends on a knowledge of the microscopic anatomy of the integument. Performing ptosis surgery without having a thorough and precise knowledge of upper lid structures would be difficult if not impossible. The evaluation of orbital tumors or orbital trauma requires an understanding of the bony structures of the orbit with its inherent weaknesses and strengths. The complex structure of the medial canthal area with its enclosed lacrimal system must be understood for one to successfully perform surgery in this area.

The skin is composed of the epidermal layer, the dermal layer, and the sub-dermal fat (Plate 2-1). The hair follicles and sebaceous glands are contained within the deeper layers of the skin. To avoid inclusion of these follicles in a skin graft, one must make the graft sufficiently thin. Or, as in cilia grafting, the graft must be deep enough to include these elements, when this is the desired effect.

The full thickness of the skin refers to all of these layers, while split thickness refers to anything less than the full thickness.

Deepithelialization provides access to the dermis and fat layers of the skin, which can be used in dermis, fat, or composite dermis-fat grafts.

Plate 2-1

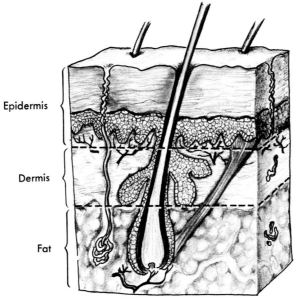

Epidermis

Dermis

Fat

Layers of skin: epidermis, dermis, fat.

Superficially the lids are composed of a layer of thin, loose skin with little subcutaneous fat. In both the upper and lower lids are transverse folds (supratarsal creases), which in the upper lid correspond approximately to the top of the tarsus.

For surgical purposes the upper lid can be divided into five layers: (1) skin, (2) orbicularis muscle, (3) orbital septum, (4) levator aponeurosis and Müller's fibers, and (5) tarsoconjunctival layer (Plate 2-2).

Underlying the skin is the orbicularis oculi, a continuous circular muscle that can be divided into orbital and palpebral parts, the latter of which is subdivided into preseptal (overlying the septum) and pretarsal (overlying the tarsus and more adherent) sections. At the lateral canthus, the pretarsal section from the upper lid joins that from the lower lid and forms the 7 mm lateral canthal tendon, which inserts on the lateral orbital tubercle. At the medial canthus, the pretarsal muscle divides into superficial and deep heads. The superficial heads unite to form the medial canthal tendon, which inserts at and nasal to the anterior lacrimal crest. The deep heads insert on the posterior lacrimal crest. Likewise, the preseptal muscle divides into superficial and deep heads, with the former inserting on the medial canthal tendon and passing to the posterior lacrimal crest, while the deep head inserts on the lacrimal diaphragm and aids in the functioning of the lacrimal pump.

The lacrimal excretory system is composed of the upper and lower puncti, with their corresponding canaliculi that descend vertically from the puncti for about 2 mm, and then course medially for 8 mm, uniting to form the common canaliculus. This empties into the lacrimal tear sac, which in turn communicates with the nose by means of the nasolacrimal duct (Plate 2-3).

The orbital septum originates from the superior orbital rim, to which it is strongly adherent.

When the mesodermally derived levator muscle advances forward in its evolution, it pushes the orbital septum in front of it and then goes on to mesh with the pretarsal orbicularis fibers and insert in the lower tarsus. The space between the septum, which finally inserts on the levator aponeurosis, and the levator itself is called the preaponeurotic space and is generally filled with fat. This is an excellent landmark during external ptosis surgery. Posterior to the levator aponeurosis is the postaponeurotic space. This space separates the aponeurosis from the smooth muscle fibers of Müller's muscle, which inserts on the tarsus.

Finally, there is the tarsal layer, about 10 mm wide in the upper lid as opposed to 4 mm wide in the lower lid. Closely adherent to the tarsus is the conjunctiva. It is this close adherence, combined with the juxtaposition of the postaponeurotic space, that makes dissection of a tarsoconjunctival flap feasible.

Plate 2-2

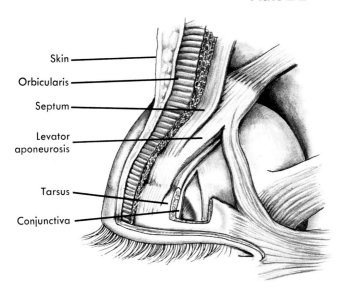

Skin
Orbicularis
Septum
Levator
aponeurosis
Tarsus
Conjunctiva

Anatomic layers of upper eyelid: skin, orbicularis muscle, septum, levator aponeurosis, tarsus, conjunctiva.

Plate 2-3

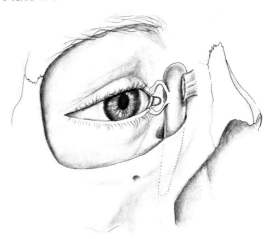

Anatomy of medial canthal area to show relationship between lacrimal excretory system and medial canthal tendon.

The orbits are generally described as four-sided conical structures, with the base forward and projecting medially toward the optic foramen.

The base, or orbital rim, is outlined by strong bony abutments: the supraorbital arch of the frontal bone above, the zygoma and maxilla below, the zygoma laterally, and the frontal process of the maxilla medially. The walls of the orbit consist of relatively thin bone.

The orbit is further divided into four parts: the roof, the medial wall, the floor, and the lateral wall.

The roof of the orbit is, for the most part, composed of the orbital plate of the frontal bone and posteriorly the lesser wing of the sphenoid (Plate 2-4, *A*). The pulley for the superior oblique muscle is lodged 4 mm behind the rim.

The medial wall, which is the thinnest of the orbital walls, is formed by the frontal process of the maxilla and the lacrimal bone, which together form the lacrimal groove (Plate 2-4, *B*). Just behind the posterior lacrimal crest is the extremely thin lamina papyracea of the ethmoids and finally the lesser wing of the sphenoid and the optic foramen.

The triangular orbital floor is formed by the zygomatic bone, the orbital process of the palatine bones, and, for the most part, the orbital plate of the maxilla, which is anterior to the infraorbital fissure. This is the area most frequently involved in blowout fractures of the orbital floor (Plate 2-4, *C*).

The lateral wall of the orbit is composed of the frontal process of the zygoma and the frontal bone anteriorly and the greater wing of the sphenoid posteriorly (Plate 2-4, *D*).

Plate 2-4

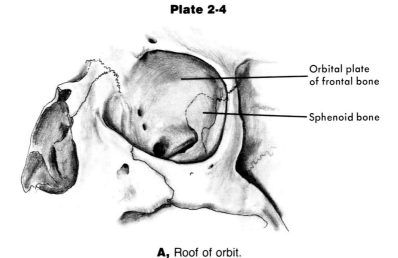

Orbital plate
of frontal bone

Sphenoid bone

A, Roof of orbit.

Plate 2-4, cont'd

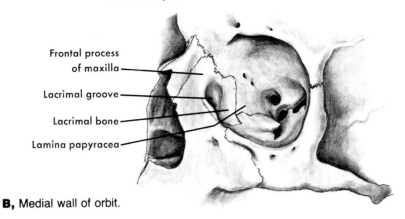

Frontal process
of maxilla

Lacrimal groove

Lacrimal bone

Lamina papyracea

B, Medial wall of orbit.

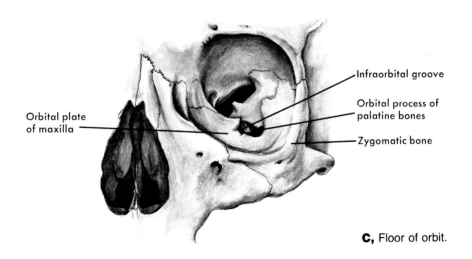

Orbital plate
of maxilla

Infraorbital groove

Orbital process of
palatine bones

Zygomatic bone

C, Floor of orbit.

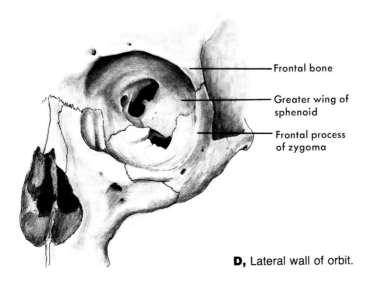

Frontal bone

Greater wing of
sphenoid

Frontal process
of zygoma

D, Lateral wall of orbit.

CHAPTER 3

SURGICAL PRINCIPLES

Although advances in the manufacture of surgical suture material, needle design and fabrication, and exquisite instrumentation have certainly increased the possibility of achieving acceptable results in all areas of surgery, including ophthalmic plastic surgery, there is no substitute for the skillful application of sound surgical principles and the sensible use of well-conceived surgical techniques in achieving successful surgical results. As previously mentioned, a precise knowledge of the regional anatomy, used to interrelate the various components of the ophthalmic complex, and a judicious and gentle handling of tissue components are required to achieve successful reconstruction.

To achieve accurate apposition of adjacent tissue layers, the correct placement and tying of sutures is essential. An inaccurately placed or inaccurately tied suture can distort the tissue margins and result in a deepened or depressed scar.

To correctly place an appositional superficial suture the wound edges should be everted. The suture should be inserted close to the wound margin and moved subcutaneously away from the margin edge. At the base of the wound, the suture should be turned and withdrawn in a similar fashion, to be inserted once again very near the edge of the opposite wound margin. The depths to which the suture is inserted on each side of the wound should be as equal as possible to prevent the formation of a depressed scar. The suture is then tied with multiple square knots and with sufficient tension to cause a slight upward puckering of the wound edges (Plate 3-1, *A*).

Placement of the suture too far from the wound edge will cause inversion of the skin margin and resultant increased cicatrization. Also, if this suture is tied too tightly, the circulation will be compromised and a delay in the healing process will result (Plate 3-1, *B*).

Plate 3-1

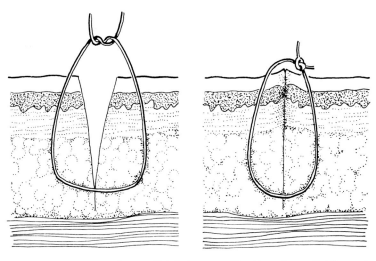

A, Correctly placed interrupted superficial closure with skin edges slightly puckered after tying.

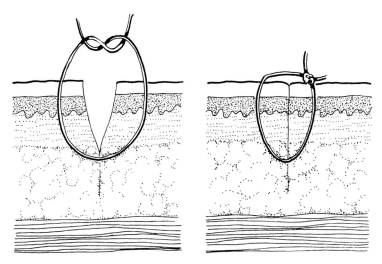

B, Incorrectly placed suture with suture too far from skin edges and inversion of margins when tied.

Deep wound
(Plates 3-2 and 3-3)

An attempt should be made to close a deep wound by the placement of a suture as near as possible to the base of the wound. If the wound is too deep for the proper placement of a single superficial suture, the deeper layers should be closed by alternate methods, with the intent of eliminating surgical dead space and the possible contracture this may cause, as well as relieving the superficial sutures of undue tension.

By simply inserting a suture in the deep layers, drawing the needle toward the surface, and reinserting the needle downward in the opposite side of the wound, the surgeon may place a buried suture with its knot turned downward (Plate 3-2, A). As many as necessary of these buried sutures are placed to relieve the tension in the skin surface. Conventional sutures are then placed on the surface.

The same effect can be achieved with a figure-of-eight suture, although the effectiveness of this suture is limited by the difficulty in its proper placement. The advantage of a properly placed figure-of-eight suture is its lack of reaction to its buried component, since this is removed with the superficial part. Removal is somewhat difficult (Plate 3-2, B).

The end-on vertical mattress suture is also useful in eliminating dead space by closure of deep tissue. The peripheral support provided by the placement of this suture also produces a good apposition of superficial wound edges. When these sutures are used, they should be alternated with simple interrupted sutures, because they tend to suppress circulation. When this suture is inserted into the underlying fascia, good apposition can also be achieved with separated underlying tissue (Plate 3-3).

Plate 3-2

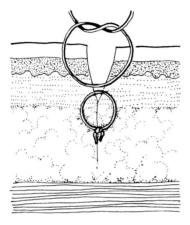

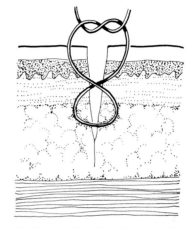

A, Buried suture used to close deeper layers. Superficial layer closed with interrupted suture.

B, Figure-of-eight suture used to achieve same closure.

Plate 3-3

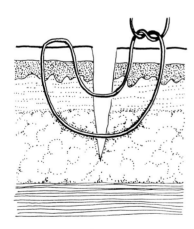

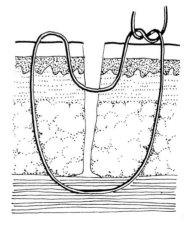

A, End-on vertical mattress suture used to eliminate dead space.

B, End-on suture used to bind superficial layer to underlying tissue.

Noncomplex lacerations
(Plates 3-4 to 3-6)

For the closure of noncomplex lacerations a time-saving and effective technique is the use of continuous locking or nonlocking sutures. If care is taken to equalize the tension along the length of suture placement, this method can produce a satisfactory wound closure. One method of placement of a continuous locking suture is demonstrated in Plate 3-4. The surgeon must decide on the appropriate technique at the time of surgery.

An alternate method of wound closure is the use of permanently buried interrupted subcutaneous sutures. Absorbable suture material is used for this horizontally placed appositional stitch. Often the wound apposition obtained makes the placement of superficial sutures unnecessary and eliminates the possiblity of epithelialization of superficial suture tracts. This suture may be placed as a continuous subcuticular stitch (Plate 3-5).

An ingenious technique of suture placement, the near-far, far-near suture is inserted into the wound superficially, near its margin, drawn across the hiatus, penetrated deeply, and withdrawn some distance (5 to 10 mm) from the skin edge (Plate 3-6, A). The suture is then reinserted on the opposite wound margin at an equidistant point, placed into the deep tissue from which it is withdrawn, and again drawn across the wound, to be withdrawn at a superficial point near the margin of the wound. The two-layered closure, of course, requires suture of sufficient strength to relieve the tension of the wound and facilitate its superficial closure (Plate 3-6, B).

Next, interrupted sutures are generally interspaced at 1 cm intervals (Plate 3-6, C). The interrupted sutures can be removed before the near-far, far-near sutures, which are generally left in place for 1 week. The wound is generally adhesively bound for several days to ensure continued wound apposition.

Plate 3-4

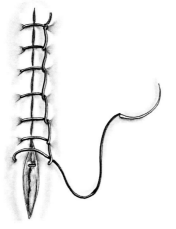

Continuous locking suture.

Plate 3-5

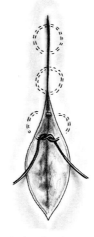

Interrupted subcutaneous sutures.

Plate 3-6

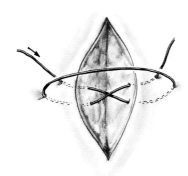

A, Near-far, far-near suture used to relieve tension.

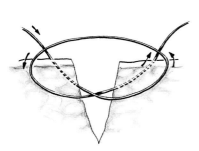

B, Directional course of near-far, far-near suture.

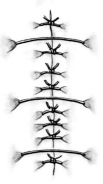

C, Placement of near-far, far-near suture interspaced with interrupted horizontal sutures.

17

USE OF FLAPS

Defects caused by traumatic injury or tumor excision that cannot be closed by direct apposition of severed tissue can be filled by the use of various skin flaps, the design of which are based on the extent, type, and location of the area to be filled.

Sliding flap   (Plate 3-7)

In some instances it is possible to undermine the tissue in a subcutaneous plane adjacent to the wound margins for a sufficient distance from the wound edge to allow tension-free closure of the defect. By repeatedly drawing together the wound edges as the dissection proceeds, one can determine when the wound will close in a tension-free fashion (Plate 3-7).

Linear advancement flap   (Plate 3-8)

A simple linear advancement flap can be used to close a rectangular defect. Parallel incisions are made from the edge of the defect, sufficiently deep to include the vascular bed and up to 2½ times the width of the area to be filled. With care taken not to compromise the circulation, the flap is gently dissected until it can be slid into the defect with minimal tension. Interrupted 6-0 silk sutures are used to close the wound.

If the length of the defect is greater than 2½ times its width, the advancement or transposition of the flap is delayed; that is, it is dissected and replaced into the donor bed for a period of 2 to 3 weeks to allow for longitudinal vascularization of the flap. At the end of this time, it is again dissected free and advanced into the recipient site (Plate 3-8).

Rotation flap   (Plate 3-9)

A rotation flap is created by incising a semicircular (curvilinear) pathway from the edge of the defect and carving a pedicle flap, again dissecting gently to include the vascular bed (Plate 3-9). The pedicle is then rotated to fill the defect. Suturing is simultaneously begun from both ends of the defect until a puckering of the curved aspect of the flap donor site is apparent. This area is then excised in a triangular fashion and the triangle is closed with interrupted sutures.

Plate 3-7

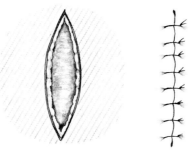

Wound margin undermined to achieve sliding flap closure.

Plate 3-8

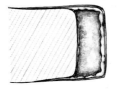 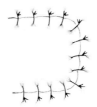

Simple linear advancement flap.

Plate 3-9

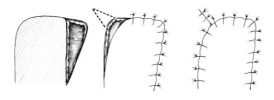

Rotation flap with triangle removed to facilitate closure.

Combined sliding and advancement flap

(Plate 3-10)

The techniques of using sliding and advancement flaps can be combined to fill a defect in which both sides of the wound need to be utilized for closure. Following the previously described methods, the flaps are created, transposed, and sutured closed (Plate 3-10).

Transposition flap

(Plate 3-11)

A transposition flap is used to close a defect in a nonadjacent area (Plate 3-11). Similar to the advancement flap, in that the flap must be delicately dissected and sufficiently thick to allow for an adequate vascular bed, this type of flap must also be gently transposed with delicate ophthalmic instruments to ensure its viability. The donor site, if unable to be closed with simple undermining of adjacent tissues, may have to be filled with an advancement flap or possibly a free skin graft, to be modified at a later date.

Plate 3-10

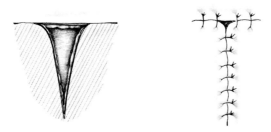

Combined sliding and advancement flap.

Plate 3-11

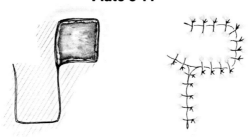

Transposition flap used to close nonadjacent defect.

A procedure essential to any ophthalmic plastic or reconstructive surgeon, Z-plasty is a relatively simple device designed to relieve a line of tension caused by a contracted scar.

The retraction of the scarred area is released by a transposition of flaps of skin whereby tissue is brought from the horizontal direction and transposed to give an increase of up to one third of the vertical length.

A central incision is made through the contracted scar, or the scar is excised. Two arm lines are then created at 60-degree angles to the central incision line (Plate 3-12, A).

Gently handling the flaps, the surgeon dissects them back so that two equal-sided triangular flaps are created. If subcutaneous scarring is present, these bands must be completely excised. Failure to release all the cicatricial bands will result in failure to release the skin flaps (Plate 3-12, B).

The flaps are then ready to be transposed (Plate 3-12, C) following this meticulous dissection of superficial skin and complete excision of fibrotic traction bands. Care must be taken to transpose the flaps in the correct direction to vertically lengthen the contracted area. We find it is far easier to close each triangle from the base to the apex; suturing is much more difficult if the apex is closed first.

The transposed flaps, when in the correct place with the scar incised or removed, will increase the vertical length of the contracted area (Plate 3-12, D).

The flaps must be dissected deep enough to include a vascular bed and to be handled without causing necrosis of the tissue. The flaps are then sutured into position with 6-0 or 7-0 silk suture (Plate 3-12, E).

Plate 3-12

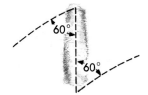

A, Central incision through line of traction with arm lines offset at 60-degree angles.

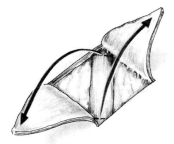

B, Flaps dissected free and elevated.

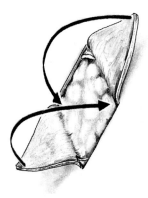

C, Fibrotic band excised and flaps ready for transposition.

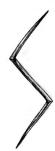

D, Flaps have been transposed.

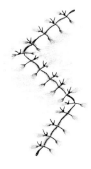

E, Flaps sutured into position.

Clinical applications

CICATRICIAL BAND

(Plate 3-13)

A cicatricial band that causes a vertical shortening of the upper lid (Plate 3-13, A) can be corrected with this technique. The contracture of the vertical scar in the central area of this lid can cause ectropion of the lid and an inability to close the eye.

A tension-relieving excision is made vertically through the scarred area of the lid. Two arms offset at 60-degree angles are then created (Plate 3-13, B) before preparation of the triangular flaps.

The flaps are carefully dissected free. The underlying scar tissue is carefully and completely excised to release the overlying contracted skin (Plate 3-13, C). Failure to completely excise the fibrotic tissue will cause a less than satisfactory result.

The flaps are then carefully transposed and placed in the proper vertical lengthening position. These flaps are sutured into place with 6-0 or 7-0 silk suture. A double-armed 6-0 silk traction suture is placed and the ends tied over a cotton or Telfa bolster (Plate 3-13, D). These are left in place for 5 days, after which time all the sutures are removed. Postoperatively the patient can benefit further from gentle massage of the previously contracted area.

Plate 3·13

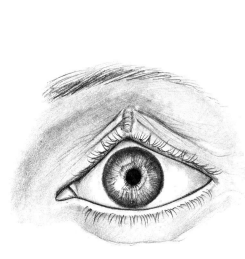

A, Cicatricial band causing vertical shortening of the upper lid.

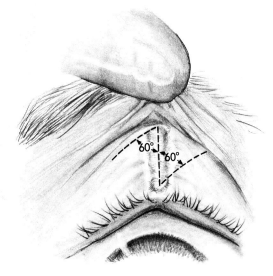

B, Central line through scar with arms offset at 60-degree angles.

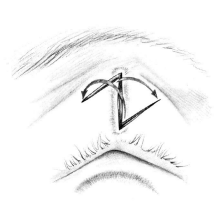

C, Flaps dissected free and ready to be transposed.

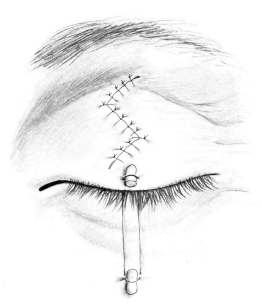

D, Flaps transposed and sutured into position with upper lid stretched.

The use of multiple Z-plasties in facial or brow scarring can be helpful in those instances in which scarring is too pronounced for dermabrasion to be used as a primary procedure. The technique follows the guidelines previously described. Following the creation of the initial incision along the length of the contracted scar (or the excision of that scar), two offset arms are created at 60-degree angles to the first incision at the extremities of the incision. Along the length of the central incision, several incisions at approximately 60-degree angles are then created as needed (Plate 3-14, *A*).

The flaps are carefully dissected and underlying fibrotic tissue excised to completely release the cutaneous layer. The arms are then carefully transposed. The flaps will virtually fall into place if the contracted bands have been adequately lysed. Interrupted 6-0 or 7-0 silk sutures are used to secure the flaps in place (Plate 3-14, *B*).

Plate 3-14

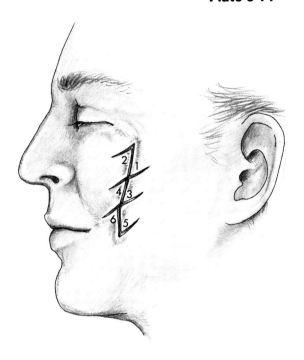

A, Multiple Z-plasty prepared.

B, Flaps carefully transposed and sutured into position.

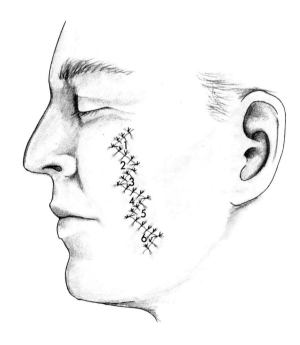

For lower lid deficiency or contracture it is possible to modify the Z-plasty technique to create a skin flap that can be used as an alternative procedure to a free skin graft.

A 4-0 silk suture is placed through the lid margin of the contracted lid and the lid stretched. An incision through skin and the fibrotic tissue is made 3 mm below the lash line and extended out to the lateral canthus. The incision is then turned medially and the central portion of the Z created with the incision ending just before reaching the supratarsal crease. The Z is completed by incising laterally to outline a temporally based flap (Plate 3-15, A). After adequate dissection to release the lower lid, with the excision of fibrotic bands, the upper triangle, having been dissected, is transposed into the lower lid defect. The upper lid and the transposition flap are sutured into place with 6-0 or 7-0 silk suture (Plate 3-15, B).

An elevation of the lateral canthus can also be corrected by an adaptation of this technique. In this case a flap of skin from the lower lid is transposed to fill a defect in the upper lid. The level of the medial canthus can be used as a guide to estimate the location of the new lateral canthus.

A central incision is created approximately 3 mm below the lash line, parallel to the lid margin, and extending from the middle of the lower lid to the lateral canthus; then the incision is turned medially and directed toward the supratarsal crease of the upper lid. The lower arm of the Z is brought temporally and ends at the desired position of the new lateral canthus (Plate 3-15, C). The lower triangular flap is gently dissected back to its base. The fibrotic tissue creating the elevation of the canthus is excised until the lateral canthus freely drops into the desired position. The lower flap is then transposed to fill the upper lid defect. Skin hooks are helpful during this type of manipulation. The wounds are closed with interrupted 6-0 or 7-0 silk sutures, which are removed after 4 to 5 days (Plate 3-15, D).

Plate 3-15

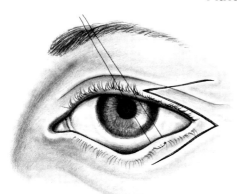

A, Z-type incision prepared to correct lower lid deficiency.

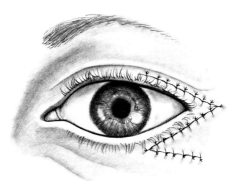

B, Upper lid flap transposed to fill deficiency and sutured into place.

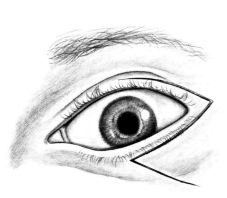

C, Central incision made along lid margin in attempt to lower lateral canthus.

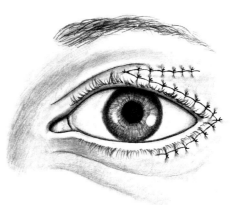

D, Lower lid flap transposed to upper lid and sutured in place.

The technique of Z-plasty can also be utilized for the correction of an elevated brow. This is a common occurrence following mismanaged traumatic lacerations, after chemical or thermal injury to the brow, or as part of a reconstructive procedure.

As in the previous procedure, the new position of the elevated brow is determined by its placement in the temporal end of the lower arm of the Z. This position can be estimated by using both the contralateral brow and the medial end of the elevated brow as landmarks. If the cilia are absent at the time of surgery, care should be taken in the placement of the transposed arm.

The central incision in this case is placed under and parallel to the cilia of the brow. The superior arm is then offset to follow the superior orbital rim (Plate 3-16, A).

The flaps are gently dissected. Care must be taken not to injure the roots of the cilia, which may nonetheless temporarily fall out.

The flaps are then transposed, with the temporal end of the lower incision receiving the extremity of the elevated brow (Plate 3-16, B).

The flaps are sutured in place with 6-0 or 7-0 silk sutures, which are left in place for 5 days.

After all of these procedures a light dressing is applied, which is changed daily for several days.

Plate 3-16

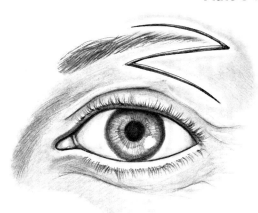

A, Correction of elevated brow by Z-type incision.

B, Transposed brow with placement at temporal end of lower arm.

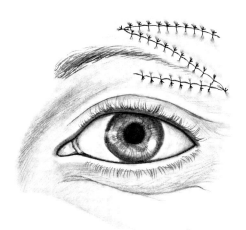

CHAPTER 4

GRAFTING TECHNIQUES

Especially useful among the various techniques in the armamentarium of the ophthalmic reconstructive surgeon are the free skin or tarsal grafts to replace scarred and contracted areas of the lids or periorbita. A knowledge of the basic procedures used in free skin grafting and several clinical applications will enable the surgeon to apply his skills in almost any case in which the use of skin grafts is indicated. Tarsal grafts are used in those cases in which the internal lamellae of the lids are shortened. They can be used alone or in combination with free skin grafts.

In Chapter 2 it was noted that the skin is divided into the epidermal layer and the dermal layer, underlying which is the subdermal fat, and that a split-thickness skin graft refers to any graft that is less than the full thickness of the skin. Inclusion of all of the layers of the skin in the graft is known as a full-thickness graft (Plate 4-1).

Full-thickness grafts are best taken from the contralateral lid, although retroauricular skin is an excellent match. If these areas are not suitable or available, split-thickness grafts may be taken from the supraclavicular or other convenient area.

The optimal area from which to take the skin graft is one that most closely matches the physical and esthetic characteristics of the site into which the graft is to be placed. A full- or split-thickness skin graft may be taken freehand or with the aid of a mechanical dermatome. We generally inject the donor site with 1% lidocaine (Xylocaine) with 1:100,000 epinephrine, even in cases in which general anesthesia is used.

Removing the epidermal layer of the skin provides access to the dermal, fat, or combined dermal-fat layers. The epidermis may be removed by dermabrasion or with a dermatome.

The dermal or dermal-fat grafts are useful for volume replacement in the facial area and for kinetic orbital implants. Removal of the dermis, fat, or dermal-fat grafts is usually done freehand and the size tailored to the area of defect to be filled.

In placing a free skin graft, a certain amount of postoperative contracture should be expected, and if possible the recipient site should be stretched or an excess of skin should be taken as a graft. Generally, about 25% of the excess should be taken as a graft. Given a suitable donor site, the graft usually blends into the adjacent skin. Occasionally, dermabrasion or minor modifications may be necessary.

Plate 4-1

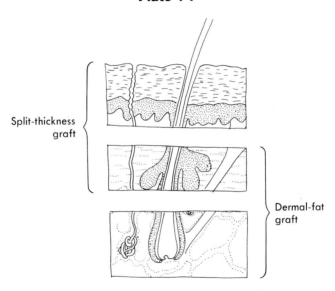

Split-thickness graft

Dermal-fat graft

Layers of integument available for grafting.

Following extensive traumatic, chemical, or thermal injury to the upper lid, a contracted scar may cause a decrease in the vertical dimension of the lid for which a simple procedure such as Z-plasty may not suffice. In these cases, a free skin graft may be needed to replace skin and fibrotic tissue that may need to be excised to release the retracted lid.

Following the placement of a 4-0 silk suture through the lid margin, an elliptical blepharoplasty-type incision is made in the upper lid. The lower incision is made parallel to the lid margin, while the upper incision forms a curved arch. The two incisions contain between them the fibrotic area to be excised (Plate 4-2, A).

Using sharp dissection, the surgeon carefully excises the contracted skin. Any underlying fibrotic bands are cut and as much as possible of the fibrotic tissue is excised to release the lid. The traction suture is used to test the elasticity of the lid. When the lid has been sufficiently released, the 4-0 silk suture is anchored to the area overlying the inferior orbital rim (Plate 4-2, B) so that the upper lid actually overrides the lower lid.

Hemostasis of the donor bed is best achieved by applying mild pressure and by vasoconstrictors, since excessive use of cautery may cause the graft to be lost.

The donor site is then selected by the criteria previously mentioned. The surgeon should accurately measure the size of the graft to be taken and should take into account the postoperative contraction that usually results. A split-thickness graft usually contracts more than a full-thickness graft.

If the contralateral upper lid is to be used as a donor site, this area is marked with a methylene blue marking pencil before the injection of the anesthetic solution (1% lidocaine with 1:100,000 epinephrine), as in an upper lid blepharoplasty (see Chapter 10). The donor material is carefully excised and gently handled. As the excision proceeds, the potential graft may be placed on a piece of Telfa dressing to aid in its handling. The skin is immediately transferred to the donor site, where it is sutured into place with 6-0 silk interrupted sutures (Plate 4-2, C).

The graft should be incised with small (1 mm) multiple full-thickness cuts to prevent fluid accumulation beneath it. A moderate Telfa pressure dressing may be tied down over it and should remain in place for several days.

The donor site may be closed as in a blepharoplasty incision, and once again cautery should be used sparingly, if at all.

If the skin from the contralateral upper lid is unavailable or proves inadequate, the retroauricular area is the next choice, followed by the supraclavicular skin. In these instances care must be taken to remove any subcutaneous fat that may be present. The retroauricular wound is closed with 4-0 silk; transient flattening of the ears occasionally may be produced.

The dressing over these grafts should be changed daily. Generally, the sutures are removed after 5 days. If the graft looks dusky after 2 days, alternate sutures should be removed.

Plate 4-2

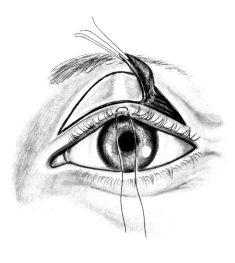

A, Excision of scar with traction suture in place.

B, Lid stretched, overriding lower lid, after fibrotic tissue excised.

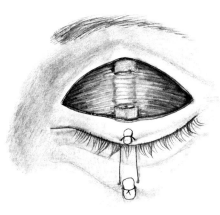

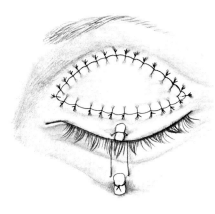

C, Full-thickness skin graft sutured in place.

In those cases in which the internal lamellae of the lower lids have been injured, a retraction and subsequent vertical shortening occurs and is evidenced by the appearance of sclera below the inferior limbus of the involved eye (Plate 4-3, *A*). Because these cases involve not only the superficial layer (for which Z-plasty would be sufficient) but also the tarsal layer, the use of a free tarsal graft taken from the ipsilateral upper lid is indicated.

Following the placement of a protective contact shell in the eye, an Erhardt clamp is placed, and the lower lid is everted. Using a razor blade knife, the surgeon makes an incision in the middle of the tarsus and extends it from the medial to the temporal aspect of the lid (Plate 4-3, *B*). The incision is carried to, but does not include, the layer of the pretarsal orbicularis. Pointed scissors are then used to spread apart the two tarsal edges of the wound, preparing a donor site and releasing the internal contracture of the lid.

The Erhardt clamp is then removed and placed on the upper lid. The lid is everted in an area 2 to 3 mm from the lid margin. A tarsal wedge is incised to approximate the size of the defect to be filled in the lower lid (Plate 4-3, *C*). On cross section, the recipient site with the separated tarsus is apparent, as is the donor site with its potential free tarsal graft (Plate 4-3, *D*).

Plate 4-3

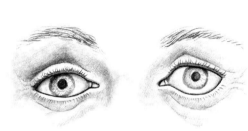

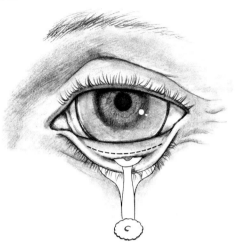

A, Vertically shortened left lower lid.

B, Midtarsal incision indicated from nasal to temporal extremity.

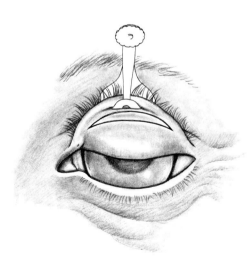

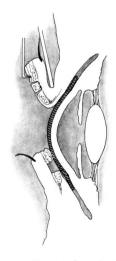

C, Everted upper lid with free tarsal graft incised.

D, Cross section to show tarsal grafts.

Next, the graft is excised from the upper lid. A sharp razor blade knife is most useful in this dissection. The excision includes conjunctiva and tarsus, but care is taken not to include the pretarsal lid structures. The 2 to 3 mm strip of tarsus near the lid margin is left to avoid causing postoperative entropion.

The tarsal graft is transferred to the recipient bed and sutured into place with fine 6-0 or 7-0 chromic catgut (Plate 4-3, *E*). These sutures may be removed after a 2-week period. The upper lid is closed with full-thickness 6-0 silk sutures. These may be removed after 5 days.

A cross-sectional view reveals the tarsal graft sutured into position and the closure of the upper lid area (Plate 4-3, *F*). An added benefit of this procedure can be the shortening of the supratarsal lid fold secondary to the placement of the full-thickness sutures.

Plate 4-3, cont'd

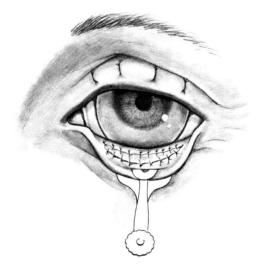

E, Tarsal graft sutured into lower lid defect.

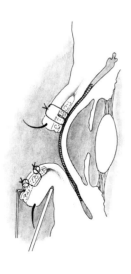

F, Cross section following procedure showing tarsal graft in place.

CHAPTER 5

LID TRAUMA

The repair of soft tissue injury to the eyelids involves the use of refined surgical and microsurgical techniques, as well as the fine technical advances that have been made in the field of instrumentation and suture production.

The initial evaluation of the injury must preclude the possibility of direct ocular injury and must include a careful slit lamp and funduscopic examination as prerequisites to evaluation of the adnexal trauma. The possibility of neurologic deficit in cases of severe trauma must be considered, with neurologic or neurosurgical consultation requested as needed.

Having ascertained that the neurologic and ocular status of the patient is normal, the surgeon turns his attention to the evaluation of the periorbita.

The area should be as carefully as possible cleansed of debris and blood. It should be ascertained if there has been tissue loss, because often the missing tissue can be located, as in windshield injuries, and a primary repair effected. (A very soft bristled toothbrush is helpful in cleaning this area.)

Following an adequate preoperative evaluation, in which the extent of tissue injury has been fully ascertained, surgical repair is begun.

Full-thickness laceration of the lid margin can be repaired using the three-suture technique. We prefer to use loupe magnification for this procedure.

A protective contact shell is used to cover the globe. Although local infiltration of 1% lidocaine with 1:100,000 epinephrine can be used, we prefer general anesthesia, because it is less disturbing to the tissues.

A razor blade knife is used to correct irregularity of the wound margin. While the medial aspect of the wound is grasped with a forceps, the razor blade knife is inserted full thickness through the lid and brought upward through the lid margin to remove any irregularities (Plate 5-1, *A*).

Next, the temporal aspect of the wound is grasped, and the razor fragment once again is inserted full thickness at the base of this apsect of the wound and brought up and through the lid margin to square the wound edge (Plate 5-1, *B*).

A double-armed 6-0 or 7-0 silk suture is used to close the wound. One end of the suture is passed through the meibomian orifice, about 1 mm from the wound margin. The other end of the suture is similarly passed through an orifice on the opposite wound margin. This suture is secured. The lid margin should be in good apposition. If it is not, the suture has been inserted at an angle and should be placed again. A second silk suture is similarly placed posterior to the first at the junction between the skin and conjunctiva and secured. The ends of these two sutures are left long, approximately 2 cm. A third lid marginal suture is placed in the lash line, with care taken not to go anterior to the lashes, because this may cause a turning in of the lid margin. The long ends of the first two sutures are tied into the knot of the third suture (Plate 5-1, *C* and *D*).

A 5-0 chromic catgut or other suitable absorbable suture is used to close the tarsal layer from the anterior side (Plate 5-1, *C*). One or more of these sutures are placed as needed. It is sometimes useful, when the lid is tense, to place one of these sutures immediately following placement of the first meibomian suture.

The orbicularis muscle usually is not closed with absorbable suture, but instead the first two or three interrupted superficial silk sutures are placed sufficiently deep to engage the severed orbicularis muscle and reapproximate it.

The remainder of the skin incision, which should be trimmed to eliminate "dog-earing," is closed with interrupted 6-0 or 7-0 silk sutures (Plate 5-1, *E*).

A light dressing is applied and should be changed daily.

The superficial sutures are removed after 3 to 4 days. The lid line sutures are left in place for 1 week.

Following removal of the lid line sutures, the lid margins should be even and regular with no notching. Although on rare occasions a small notch will fill in adequately, excision of the notch and reanastomosis is generally required.

Plate 5-1

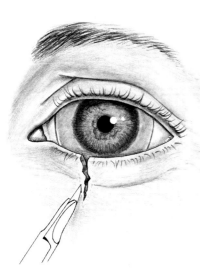

A, Razor blade knife used to correct irregularity of medial aspect of wound.

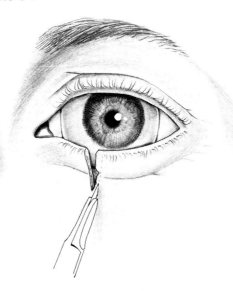

B, Temporal aspect of wound similarly treated.

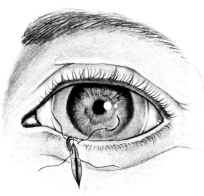

C, Long ends of central and posterior sutures tied through lash line suture. Tarsus closed with absorbable suture.

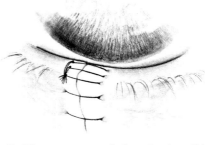

D, Three-suture technique to close lid margin.

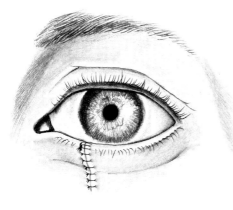

E, Interrupted sutures used to close skin incision.

The integrity of the lacrimal drainage system must be reestablished after transmarginal lacerations that involve the canaliculi in the area between the punctum and the medial canthus (Plate 5-2, *A*).

Although most patients with a single functioning canaliculus remain asymptomatic, some have severe epiphora. Therefore one should always attempt a repair as near as possible to the time of injury.

A variety of methods have been attempted to effect a repair of these canalicular injuries. The method that seems to give the most consistent results is monocanalicular intubation of the severed duct, combined with its direct anastomosis.

Since a transmarginal laceration is generally associated with these injuries, this wound is repaired simultaneously by the previously mentioned techniques. Before the previously placed marginal sutures are secured, a piece of polyethylene tubing is inserted through the severed canaliculus and out the punctum. One can usually locate the ends of the canaliculus with the aid of the operating microscope. With the tubing in place, the duct is sutured with 10-0 nylon or 8-0 absorbable suture. The suture in the marginal laceration is then secured. The loose end of the polyethylene tubing is sutured to the skin of the lower lid and taped into place (Plate 5-2, *B*).

Plate 5-2

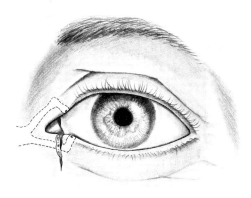

A, Full-thickness lid laceration involving lower canaliculus.

B, Monocanalicular intubation of severed canaliculus.

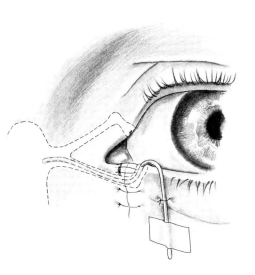

An alternative method is the insertion of a piece of polyethylene tubing within the severed canaliculus with the subsequent closure of the duct and transmarginal laceration over it (Plate 5-3). The disadvantage of this procedure is the eventual irritation that the presence of this device causes within the delicate canaliculus.

Although many surgeons currently think that it is wise not to disturb a functioning canaliculus in the repair of a severed one, it is possible to repair a severed duct by inserting the microtubing through the upper canaliculus and out the lower one. A suture is then threaded through the lumen of the tubing and tied. The suture is rotated so that the potentially irritating knot is within the tube. Next, the tube is rotated so that only smooth surfaces come into contact with traumatized or delicate structures (Plate 5-4, *A*).

In a somewhat different version of this procedure, a longer piece of microtubing is threaded through both canaliculi and made to exit through the nasolacrimal duct into the nose, where it is cuffed (Plate 5-4, *B*). The tubing should not be pulled too tightly, because it can erode the punctum.

The superficial suture is removed after 4 days, while the transmarginal sutures can remain for 1 week. The stint should be left in place for 4 to 6 weeks.

Plate 5-3

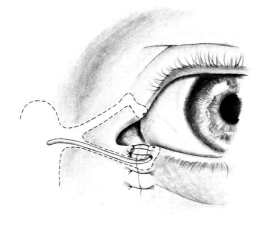

Polyethylene tubing within canaliculus.

Plate 5-4

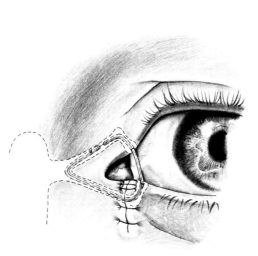

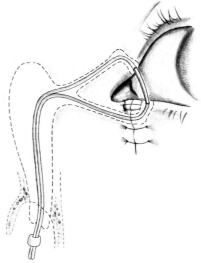

A, Bicanalicular intubation with suture threaded within.

B, Bicanalicular intubation with ends of tubing through nasolacrimal duct.

The superficial heads of the pretarsal muscle unite to form the medial canthal tendon. Often in transmarginal lacerations involving the canaliculus, the superficial heads forming the canthal tendon are severed and difficult to locate.

A simple method of locating these structures is to make a vertical incision over the insertion of the medial canthal tendon and dissect down to its periosteal insertion (Plate 5-5, *A*). It is often helpful to inject the area with 1% lidocaine with 1:100,000 epinephrine before making the incision.

A blunt scissors is used to trace the course of the superficial heads of the pretarsal orbicularis back to the point at which they are severed (Plate 5-5, *B*). These are anastomosed directly with 5-0 chromic catgut (Plate 5-5, *C*). (This incision is also indicated in injuries directly involving the medial canthal tendon.) The canaliculi and transmarginal laceration are then closed as previously described. The incision over the medial canthal tendon is closed with interrupted 6-0 silk sutures (Plate 5-5, *D*).

Plate 5-5

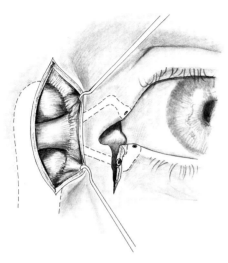

A, Canalicular laceration combined with laceration of medial canthal tendon. Insertion of medial canthal tendon exposed.

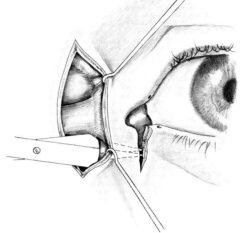

B, Dissection carried through to distal side of severed tendon.

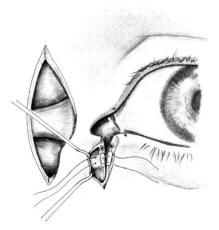

C, Anastomosis of severed canthal tendon.

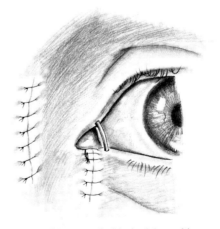

D, Closure of skin incision with canalicular tubing in place.

CHAPTER 6

EXCISION OF MARGINAL LID TUMORS

The variability in the presentation of malignant marginal lid tumors often makes the diagnosis a difficult one, and therefore any lesion of the lid margin that leaves even a modicum of doubt in the surgeon's mind should be sent for microscopic diagnosis.

EXCISIONAL BIOPSY

Although the history of the evolution of a lid mass can be useful to the surgeon and even though serial photography can be used to follow its progression, we generally prefer the simple certainty of an excisional biopsy of these tumors to ensure peace of mind—both to the patient and to the surgeon.

Raised lesion   (Plate 6-1)

The type of excisional biopsy we perform depends on the shape, size, and location of the lesion that is present. For raised lesions of the lid margin, we generally prefer a direct knife blade excision at the lid margin.

If the biopsy is performed as an office procedure in a minor surgical setting, the lid is prepared and draped in the usual fashion and anesthetized with 2% lidocaine with 1:100,000 epinephrine to provide lid akinesia and to ensure hemostasis. The surgeon uses a gloved fingertip as a backguard (Plate 6-1) to provide protection for the globe down to the cul-de-sac and as a rigid base for the lower lid. A sharp knife or razor blade fragment is used to excise this tumor mass at its base, leaving a smooth and level lid margin. The blade is directed toward the fingertip so that this can facilitate the excision by the firmness it provides the lid. As large a piece as possible, if not all of the mass, is excised.

Inferiorly directed lesion   (Plate 6-2)

For inferiorly directed lesions the blade of the knife is turned in the opposite direction (Plate 6-2) and with the same sawing motion, this time away from the globe, the lesion is excised, with care to leave the lash roots intact, in the event that the lesion is benign.

Plate 6-1

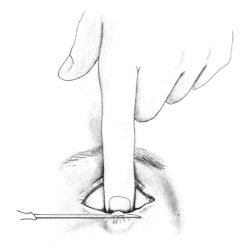

Knife blade used to excise a raised lesion.

Plate 6-2

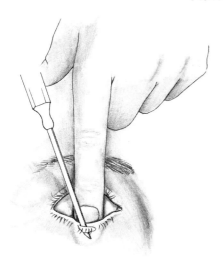

Lash roots left in place as inferiorly directed lesion is excised.

Flat lesion (Plate 6-3)

In those cases involving a flat lesion of the lid margin, a fingertip or bone plate is again inserted down to the inferior fornix. The lid is prepared and draped in the usual manner and infiltrated with a local anesthetic, as described previously. A sharp knife or razor blade is used to perforate the mass at the lateral lid margin (Plate 6-3, *A*). The incision is carried to the medial extremity of the mass (Plate 6-3, *B*).

The medial end of the lesion is then cut free (Plate 6-3, *C*) and grasped with a toothed forceps while the knife blade is reversed and used to excise the tumor mass completely (Plate 6-3, *D*).

Frequently, light cautery is used to control bleeding from the wound edge if moderate pressure fails to achieve hemostasis.

Plate 6-3

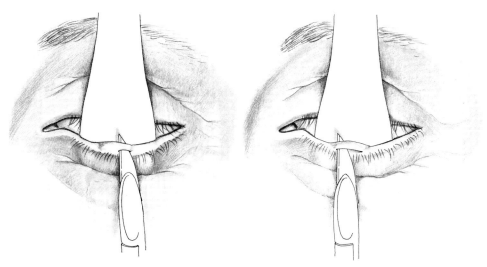

A, Razor blade perforates flat lesion at lateral extremity.

B, Lesion incised to medial extremity.

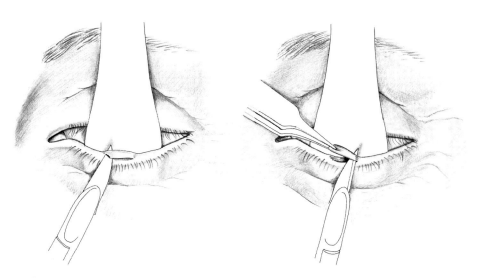

C, Medial edge of lesion cut free.

D, Excision of lesion being completed.

Dermabrasion is also a useful technique that can be employed for the removal of small benign lesions or scars of the lid margin.

Once again, the lid should be adequately prepared and draped and the area infiltrated with a local anesthetic.

With the fingertip or other rigid instrument behind the lid, a piece of sandpaper wrapped around the fingertip can be used to abrade superiorly placed lid masses (Plate 6-4, *A*), as well as those on the anterior lid surface (Plate 6-4, *B*).

A mechanical dermabrader can also be used to remove these lesions, often with less effort than the manual method, although certainly a manually operated device avoids the apparent unreliability of the mechanical devices (Plate 6-4, *C*).

Plate 6-4

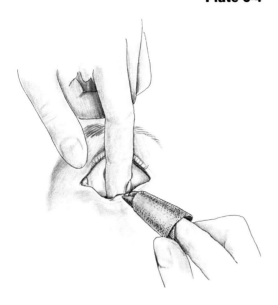

A, Fine sandpaper used to level tumor mass.

B, Sandpaper used to level mass on anterior lid edge.

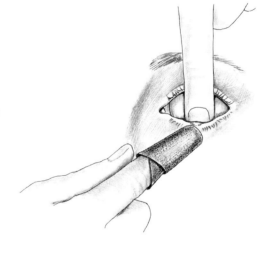

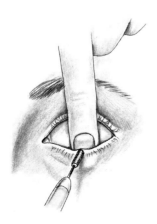

C, Mechanical dermabrader used to level lid mass.

If the lesion is found to be malignant, as in the case of a basal cell carcinoma, an en bloc resection of the involved area is performed (Plate 6-5, *A*).

When excising malignant lesions of the lids, we generally prefer the excision that will ensure complete elimination of the tumor mass, giving thought to reconstruction of the lid only after the tumor is completely excised. One of the major causes of recurrence of malignant lid tumors is failure to completely eradicate the lesion at the primary surgery because of apprehension at the thought of a major reconstruction.

Preoperatively the surgeon should try to ascertain the limits of the lesion by transillumination of the lid margin of the involved area. In the presence of a malignancy the meibomian gland orifices are obliterated or deranged. It is usually necessary to go beyond the abnormal architecture by two to three meibomian orifices to ensure complete elimination of the tumor (Plate 6-5, *B*).

After the en bloc specimen has been excised, 1 mm marginal and basal sections should be removed and appropriately labeled (Plate 6-5, *C*). If facilities for frozen sections are available, these should be examined at the time of surgery. The surgeon must realize that the appearance of tumor in only part of the marginal section necessitates further excision in that area.

Finally, the lid defect is closed by the three-suture technique, as has been previously described (Plate 6-5, *D* and *E*). If a more extensive excision has been necessary, a reconstructive procedure will be needed.

Plate 6-5

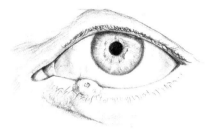

A, Malignant lesion occupying medial one third of lower lid.

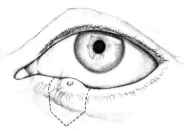

B, Margin of excision extends two to three normal meibomian orifices beyond lesion.

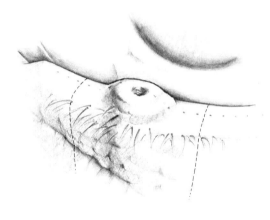

C, Area to be excised with marginal and basal sections slated for excision.

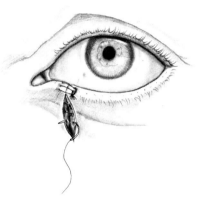

D, Closure of lid defect with three-suture technique.

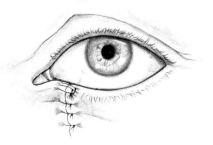

E, Lid defect sutured closed.

CHAPTER 7

EYELID RECONSTRUCTION

The surgeon who performs ophthalmic plastic surgery of the ocular adnexa should be familiar with a series of reconstructive procedures that would enable him to successfully repair eyelid defects, beginning with a simple lid-laceration type of closure and progressing to the repair of areas of appreciable tissue loss, as in cases of large medial canthal carcinomas.

The surgeon's ability to perform this type of surgery is based on an accurate knowledge of the normal regional anatomy combined with a proficiency in the fundamental principles and techniques in ophthalmic plastic surgery that have already been described. In addition, the surgeon should have in mind a stepwise plan for solving increasingly complex reconstructive problems based on the size and location of the defect.

Since a primary closure cannot always be effected, the surgeon should be prepared to employ lid-lengthening procedures such as lateral canthotomy and cantholysis and proceed to composite grafts and lateral advancement flaps when these fail. In the event that even more tissue is required for reconstruction, he should be familiar with the use of tarsoconjunctival flaps, bridge flaps, transposition flaps, lined pedicle flaps, and Mustardé-type techniques for lower and upper lid use. Because of the very unusual anatomy of the canthi, the procedures and principles described here are unique and need to be learned.

A deficiency in the horizontal dimension of the eyelid, whether it is traumatic, congenital, or iatrogenic (for example, following tumor excision) is termed a coloboma if it involves less than the entire lid.

Generally, the type of closure is the same as that for a transmarginal laceration, unless the defect is of such a magnitude that a lid-lengthening or other more complex reconstructive procedure is needed.

Because of the rounded edges of a congenital or long-standing traumatic coloboma, the margins of the defect need to be excised so that the wound edges can be anastomosed.

In general, an attempt should be made to create a pentagon-shaped defect (Plate 7-1, *A*), which will provide a smooth and regular lid closure.

Following the placement of a protective contact shell over the globe, a local anesthetic is injected if general anesthesia is not employed. The margin of the defect, which in most congenital cases is in the nasal aspect of the upper lid, is grasped and a razor blade knife used to create a smooth raw edge, excising even the benign dermoids that are occasionally present (Plate 7-1, *B*).

Using the near-far, far-near technique, the surgeon passes a 4-0 silk suture through the lid and tarsus. This will permit closure of a moderately large defect, although it may cause a ptosis, which would require later correction (Plate 7-1, *C*).

With the wound edges in apposition, the lid margin is closed with the three-suture technique, and the tarsal layer is closed with interrupted 5-0 chromic catgut or other suitable absorbable suture. The overlying skin is closed with interrupted 6-0 silk sutures (Plate 7-1, *D*).

A light dressing is applied. Superficial sutures are removed after 4 days and marginal sutures 3 days later.

Plate 7-1

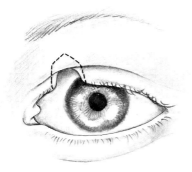

A, Coloboma of nasal aspect of upper lid.

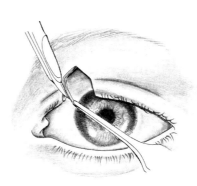

B, Marginal tissues excised to create pentagonal shape.

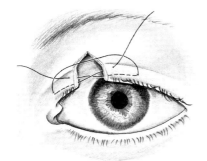

C, Near-far, far-near suture placed.

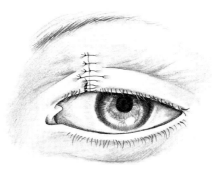

D, Lid margin and cutaneous sutures placed.

In closing defects too large for direct transmarginal suturing, it is possible to relax the tension of the lid by means of a lateral canthotomy; this is performed with scissors after crushing the tissue with a hemostat (Plate 7-2, *A*). A forceps or a mattress suture can be used to draw the wound edges together, thus enabling the surgeon to ascertain if the tension on the lid will necessitate this procedure.

If the defect is somewhat larger, an additional relaxation of the lid can be obtained by lysis of the lower crus of the lateral canthal tendon. With a Westcott scissors, skin is dissected away from the lower crus anteriorly, while the conjunctiva is stripped away posteriorly (Plate 7-2, *B*). The isolated lower crus of the tendon is then severed, with care taken not to injure the superior crus (Plate 7-2, *C*).

The lysis of this inferior crus of the lateral canthal tendon will allow the mobilization of perhaps 5 mm of the lateral aspect of the lower lid, which can now be swung medially (Plate 7-2, *D*).

The lid margin is closed by the three-suture technique, with absorbable sutures used to close the tarsus and 6-0 silk suture used to close the superficial area. The lateral canthal area can be sutured with 6-0 absorbable suture (Plate 7-2, *E*).

A light dressing is applied; it is removed on the first postoperative day. The superficial sutures are removed after 4 days and the lid margin sutures 3 days later.

Plate 7-2

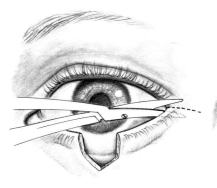

A, Lateral canthotomy performed.

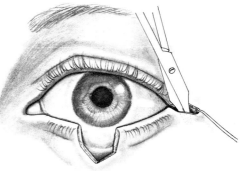

B, Skin and orbicularis incised to reveal lateral canthal tendon.

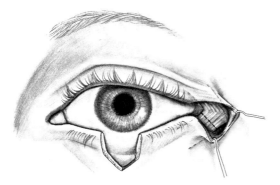

C, Exposed lower crus of lateral canthal tendon.

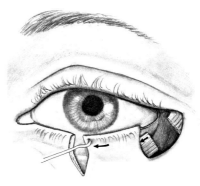

D, Tendon incised and temporal aspect of lid released.

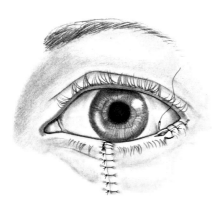

E, Lid margin and skin incision closed. Lateral canthal area closed.

When a lid defect is of such a magnitude that a tension-free closure cannot be achieved even following lateral cantholysis, it is possible to effect the closure by means of a composite graft. A composite graft, such as a full-thickness eyelid graft, contains within it multiple tissue elements.

A large central defect of the upper lid can be closed by utilizing this technique. Following lateral cantholysis in the recipient lid, the size of the donor graft that is needed for closure is estimated and outlined on the contralateral lid. By digitally compressing this lid, the surgeon can estimate the potential for use as a donor (Plate 7-3, *A*).

A lateral cantholysis can also be performed in the donor lid to better estimate its donor potential and facilitate closure following the removal of the free graft.

Following the insertion of a protective contact shell over the globe, suitable akinesia is obtained (although general anesthesia is preferred for this procedure).

A blunt scissors is used to make a full-thickness incision in the donor lid perpendicular to the lid margin and angled to form half of a pentagon. The margins of the wound are overlapped to ensure that closure will be possible following the excision. The pentagonal wedge is then excised.

The donor site is closed as a transmarginal laceration by using the three-suture technique, and the graft is transferred to the recipient lid (Plate 7-3, *B*).

To orient the graft in its recipient bed, two sutures are placed in the pretarsal orbicularis (Plate 7-3, *C*). The graft is sutured into place, with 6-0 chromic catgut used to close the subcutaneous layer and 6-0 or 7-0 silk used to close the skin (Plate 7-3, *D*).

These grafts are extremely delicate and should be handled gently. The superficial sutures should not be tied too tightly. The subcutaneous sutures should be meticulously placed so as to approximate the tarsus and the marginal wounds closed with the three-suture technique. No dressings are applied.

Plate 7-3

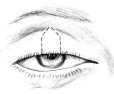 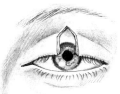

A, Large central defect in left upper lid with area of composite graft outlined on right upper lid.

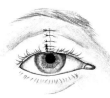 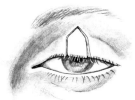

B, Graft placed in defect of left upper lid. Right upper lid closed with three-suture technique.

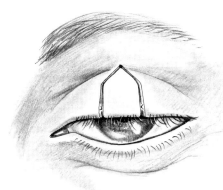 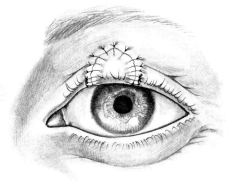

C, Graft with pretarsal fascial suture in place.

D, Graft sutured in place.

Composite graft with pedicle flap

A composite graft may also be taken from an opposing lid with a small attached pedicle retained. The usefulness of pedicles is probably more theoretic than real, since they are extremely fragile and often slough as a result of pressure necrosis from even a mild insult. For this reason, all but the lightest of dressings are avoided in composite grafting.

The donor site from which these grafts are taken is located either temporally or nasally to the defect (Plate 7-4, *A*).

Following the same technique of lateral cantholysis, the donor graft is incised and rotated gently to fill the defect (Plate 7-4, *B*). The pedicle flap is carefully sutured into place and the donor site closed by the same suture techniques as for the free graft (Plate 7-4, *C*).

The pedicle is lysed after a 2- to 3-week interval.

Plate 7-4

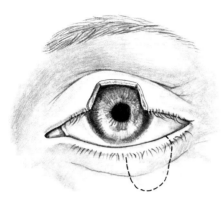

A, Central lid defect with lower lid pedicle flap outlined.

B, Pedicle flap rotated to fill defect.

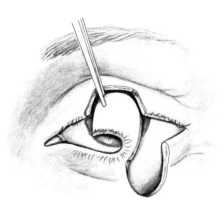

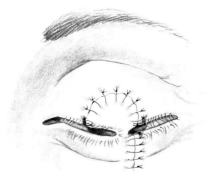

C, Pedicle flap sutured into defect and lower lid donor site closed.

Useful for reconstruction of defects in both the upper and lower lids, semicircular temporal advancement flaps permit the mobilization of additional lid substance without the necessity of using delicate composite grafts, which disturb an otherwise normal lid. Similar to other types of sliding grafts from the lateral canthus used in this type of reconstruction, this procedure offers the advantage of minimizing the horizontal dissection of the temporal area with less possibility of scarring. It can be used to fill central defects of up to one half the length of the lid.

Following the placement of a protective contact shell over the globe, the lateral canthal area is suitably anesthetized. The lid defect is trimmed to ensure smooth wound margins and a pentagonal slope. A skin-orbicularis flap is carved beginning at the lateral canthus and extending superiorly and temporally in a crescentic shape (Plate 7-5, A). The surgeon opens the lateral canthus by means of performing a canthotomy, and the inferior crus of the lateral canthal tendon is lysed.

Viable and healthy conjunctiva from the original defect can be conserved as a lining for the flap. Or, if the surgeon chooses, a free tarsal graft from the upper lid or a mucous membrane graft may be used as a lining. It may be necessary to excise a triangular piece of skin at the base of the flap to prevent puckering.

If the tissues have been adequately freed, the lateral portion of the lid can be freely rotated and advanced to fill the central defect.

The central wound is closed with the three-suture technique, as previously described. The lateral canthus is closed with a vertical mattress suture, the deep part of which passes full thickness through the upper lid substance and joins it to the full thickness of the lower lid tissue; the suture then unites the new lower lid to the original canthal angle. This suture is tightly secured. The remainder of the wound is closed with near-far, far-near sutures interspersed with 6-0 interrupted sutures (Plate 7-5, B).

A light dressing is applied. Superficial sutures are removed after 4 days; the lid margin, mattress, and near-far, far-near sutures are removed 3 days later.

Plate 7-5

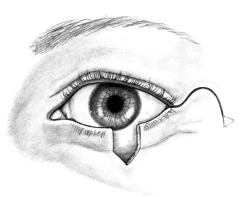

A, Semicircular skin-orbicularis flap carved at lateral canthus.

B, Lid defect closed with three-suture technique and lateral canthus closed with near-far, far-near sutures.

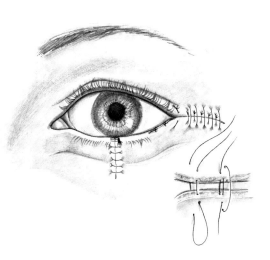

For the reconstruction of large central defects of the lower eyelid, the use of a tarsoconjunctival flap advanced from the opposing upper lid is a most satisfactory procedure. The graft serves as the inner lamella of the lid, and a skin-orbicularis flap from the cheek can serve as a superficial layer if there is adequate skin laxity.

Alternatively, a free skin graft can be used to cover the flap in those cases in which there is not adequate skin for advancement.

Following the placement of a contact shell in the eye, adequate lid akinesia should be achieved by the use of 2% lidocaine with 1:100,000 epinephrine, although general anesthesia is preferred in these cases because of the extensive dissection and the need not to distort the tissue.

The lower lid defect is trimmed to give smooth edges to the wound, with the surgeon sacrificing as little viable tissue as possible. In cases in which there is sufficient laxity of cheek skin, a methylene blue pencil is used to outline the area of the superficial advancement flap to include two relaxing triangles at the base (Plate 7-6, *A*).

The desired flap is carved from the tarsus and conjunctiva of the upper lid in the potential plane that exists between Müller's muscle and the levator aponeurosis (Plate 7-6, *B*).

The upper lid is everted on an Erhardt clamp; 3 mm below the lash line a razor blade incision is made through the conjunctiva and the tarsus parallel to the lid margin. The rim of the tarsus must be preserved to prevent postoperative entropion. In earlier literature, splitting of the lid substance was advocated, but upper lid defects resulted and an otherwise normal lid was injured. Obviously, a healthy upper lid is a prerequisite for this procedure.

The tarsoconjunctival flap is then cut with a Westcott scissors to a width that would fill the defect with a slight stretching to prevent flaccidity in the newly formed lid. The perpendicular incisions should be extended high into the fornix. The dissection should be continued so that eventually the graft falls easily into the lower part of the defect. If the flap is not dissected sufficiently into the fornix, arching of the donor lid will result.

Following removal of the contact shell, the lower end of the flap is sutured with 6-0 chromic catgut suture to the remaining conjunctiva of the lower lid. The lateral aspects of the lower lid wound are then grooved at the mucocutaneous junction to receive the edges of the flap (Plate 7-6, *C*).

A double 6-0 silk suture is passed in vertical mattress fashion from the conjunctival aspect of the grooves, through the tarsal graft, and then through the interior leaf of the groove to pull the sides of the graft into position when they are tied (Plate 7-6, *D*). The skin in the inferior triangles is excised at this point.

Plate 7-6

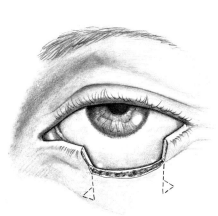

A, Large central defect with outline of external advancement flap.

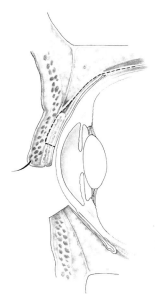

B, Sagittal section demonstrating outline of advancement flap.

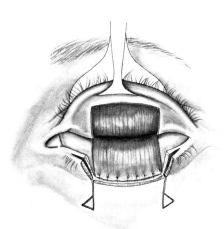

C, Everted lid with advancement flap dissected and sutured into defect. Lower lid grooves created to receive edges of flap.

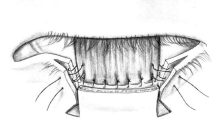

D, Insertion of mattress suture to pull tarsus into grooves.

The mattress sutures are tied over suitable bolsters; we prefer cotton. The skin-orbicularis flap is then advanced superiorly. The flap should be sufficiently dissected so that no vertical shortening of the external lamella occurs. If the cheek skin is insufficient for adequate closure, a free graft must be employed. The edge of the inferior flap is brought into line with the lid margin and sutured to the anterior aspect of the tarsoconjunctival graft with 6-0 silk sutures. Extreme care must be taken to not injure the underlying cornea. The superficial wounds are closed with interrupted 6-0 silk suture (Plate 7-6, *E*). The upper lid hangs freely over the advanced graft and need not be disturbed in any way (Plate 7-6, *F*).

We prefer to use a light dressing over these wounds. Telfa covered with loose gauze is sufficient. Dressings are changed daily for several days. The superficial sutures can be removed after 4 to 5 days. The mattress sutures are removed after 1 week.

A free skin graft, if needed, can be taken from the contralateral upper lid or other suitable area. If skin from the ipsilateral upper lid is used, a vertical shortening will result. The graft is sutured with 6-0 silk sutures placed at 1 mm intervals. It should contain multiple stab incisions for drainage and an adequate bolster. If the graft appears dusky postoperatively, alternate sutures can be removed for drainage (Plate 7-6, *G*).

The tarsorrhaphy can be opened after 4 to 6 weeks. A protective instrument is inserted beneath the flap and a blunt scissors used to incise the graft (Plate 7-6, *H*). The margin of the lower lid is leveled. The tissue of the upper lid retracts into position and need not be sutured.

At one time, cilia grafting was performed to complete this procedure, but recently we have found that artificial lashes produce an excellent cosmetic result without the possibility of postoperative complications of the cilia graft.

Plate 7-6, cont'd

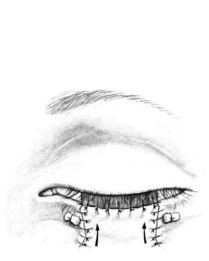

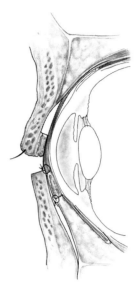

E, Advancement of external flap to cover graft.

F, Sagittal view of tarsoconjunctival flap covered with advancement flap.

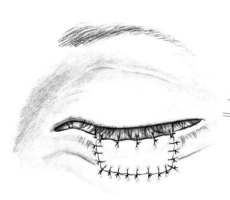

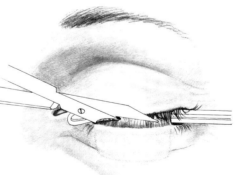

G, Free skin graft used in place of advancement flap.

H, Opening of tarsorrhaphy.

A full-thickness bridge flap can be utilized for repairing large central defects of the upper lid.

As we have seen, the techniques of lateral canthotomy and cantholysis, composite grafting, and semicircircular advancement flaps can all be used for the repair of upper lid defects. However, when the defect is so large that even the combination of more than one of these procedures is insufficient, we prefer the bridge flap over those procedures that require rotation flaps hinged on a narrow pedicle. This involves the full substance of the lower lid in preference to procedures using horizontal advancement flaps of the lateral canthal area, which are better suited for lower lid repair.

Following the injection of suitable anesthetic in the lid, when for some reason general anesthesia cannot be used, the full-thickness upper lid defect is trimmed to ensure smooth edges while sacrificing as little as possible of the healthy lid tissue. A methylene blue marking pencil is used to delineate a base-down flap 3 mm below the lash line. The width of the flap should be the size of the defect to be filled (Plate 7-7, *A*).

With a bone plate or other suitable lid clamp behind the lower lid, the anterior surface of the flap is incised over the marked area. Care must be taken to remain 3 mm from the lash line so as not to damage the marginal arterial arcade. The incision should include skin alone (Plate 7-7, *B*). The lid is everted and a separate incision made through conjunctiva and tarsus to be in apposition with the anterior incision. A Westcott scissors is used to connect the two incisions. This is done to avoid angling the flap edge, which may cause damage to the arterial arcade.

The surgeon uses the scissors to extend the dimensions of the flap horizontally until the desired width is achieved. From the ends of the incision, full-thickness vertical incisions are created down to the lower fornix. Both the flap and the bridge must be handled gently to avoid compromising the circulation. It is useful to handle the bridge by means of thin, soft rubber tubing passed under it rather than with instruments.

The bridge flap, freed from any attachments on three sides, is now gently passed under the marginal bridge. The conjunctiva and Müller's fibers of the upper lid are sutured to the conjunctiva of the advancement flap with 6-0 chromic sutures (Plate 7-7, *C*). The levator aponeurosis and septal layer of the upper lid are joined to the orbicularis of the flap with 6-0 absorbable sutures. The skin wound is closed with interrupted 6-0 silk sutures. Therefore the flap passes under the marginal bridge and extends upward to join the base of the defect in the upper lid, where it is anastomosed (Plate 7-7, *D*). The posterior surface of the flap protects the eye.

Plate 7-7

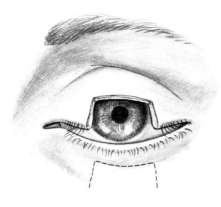

A, Large central upper lid defect with outline of full-thickness donor flap.

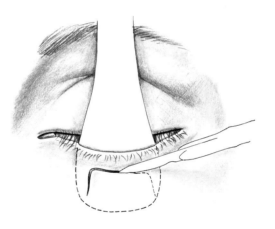

B, Lid plate in position as external incision of flap is created.

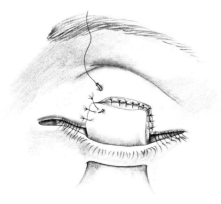

C, Advancement flap passed beneath lid margin bridge and sutured into defect.

The inferior edge of the bridge flap is left to reepithelialize on its own, with no sutures used, to avoid undue pressure.

A Telfa strip, with an appropriate area for the bridge removed, is applied and covered with a light gauze dressing. Superficial sutures are removed after 4 to 5 days.

Following a 4- to 6-week interval, during which time the flap stretches to almost double its length (Plate 7-7, *E*), the tarsorrhaphy is opened. A protective instrument is placed under the flap, and it is incised with a knife blade (Plate 7-7, *F*).

The lower edge of the newly created lid will epithelialize on its own. The lower edge of the marginal bridge is denuded and sutured to the upper edge of the skin flap. Cilia grafting has now been abandoned by us in favor of artificial lashes.

The lower lid should be in the original position with no vertical deficit, and the upper lid should be of good contour (Plate 7-7, *G*).

Plate 7-7, cont'd

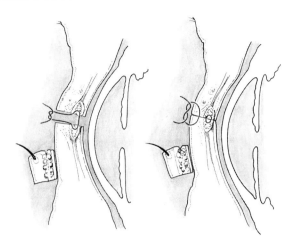

D, Sagittal section of advancement flap under marginal bridge with sutures in place.

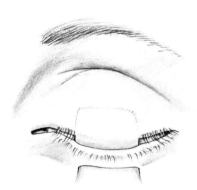
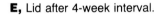

E, Lid after 4-week interval.

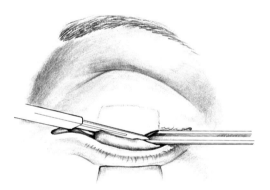

F, Tarsorrhaphy being opened after 6 weeks.

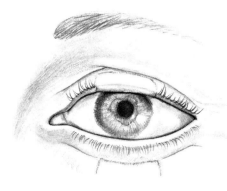

G, Lid position 6 months after surgery.

A procedure that is particularly suited for replacement of an entire upper lid, the Mustardé technique is one that requires considerable experience in the technique and handling of large dissections. The ophthalmologist who does not have the skill and training to perform such procedures should probably call on the expertise of a surgeon trained in facial plastic work. A poor result with this procedure means considerable facial distortion and potential loss of both upper and lower lids. This procedure is presented here so that the surgeon will have some familiarity with the handling of as extensive a problem as complete upper lid loss.

General anesthesia is usually preferred with this procedure because of the extent of the dissection.

A curvilinear incision is begun at the lateral canthus, arching superiorly and temporally and then down in front of the ear. The lower crus of the lateral canthal tendon is then released. A skin muscle dissection is completed so that the cheek flap is ready for rotation. Just temporal to the punctum, a full-thickness lid incision is made into the lower fornix, and the entire lower lid is used at the level of the inferior orbital rim, with a small pedicle left attached at the lateral canthus. The area below the excised lid is carved into a triangular shape (Plate 7-8, *A*).

A piece of nasal septal cartilage is then obtained. The cartilage obtained should have nasal mucosa on one side of it. The cartilage is trimmed to fill the inner lamellar defect now present in the lower lid. The mucosal side of the graft faces the globe. The remaining conjunctiva in the lower lid is sutured with 6-0 chromic catgut sutures to the mucosa. The cartilage is secured to the remaining tarsus laterally and to orbicularis inferiorly with 5-0 chromic catgut sutures (Plate 7-8, *B*).

The cheek flap is then rotated medially and the lower eyelid brought into position to fill the upper lid defect (Plate 7-8, *C*). The pedicle must be treated gently, because it contains the marginal artery needed for survival of the flap. The conjunctival layer (nasal mucosa) of the new lower lid is sutured with 6-0 chromic sutures to the edge of the cheek flap. The cheek flap is closed with 6-0 silk sutures.

In the new upper lid the conjunctiva of the flap is sutured to the conjunctiva of the defect with fine absorbable sutures. The levator, septum, and orbicularis are approximated to the flap structures. The skin is closed with 6-0 silk interrupted sutures.

A light dressing is applied to avoid necrosis to the pedicle. Superficial sutures are removed after 4 to 5 days. The pedicle is severed after 3 weeks and the lid margins are revised (Plate 7-8, *D*).

Plate 7-8

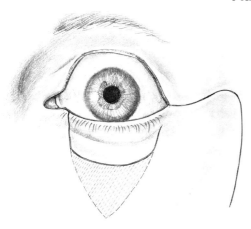

A, Deficiency of entire upper lid with dissection of temporal curvilinear rotation flap and release of entire lower lid.

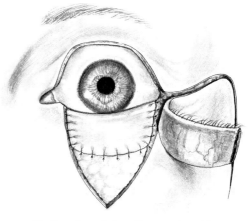

B, Nasal septal cartilage sutured in place of tarsoconjunctival flap.

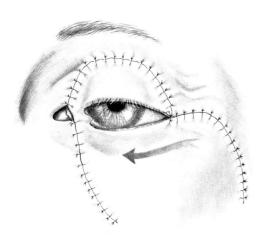

C, Curvilinear flap rotated nasally while lower lid transposed superiorly.

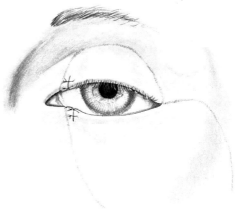

D, Interpalpebral band lysed and lid margin revised.

Temporal advancement flaps are suitable as a means of lower lid replacement and, if the defect is small enough, can be used without replacing the inner lamella of the lid. However, the usual reason for using this type of flap is that the defect is of such a magnitude that simpler and more direct means of lid closure are insufficient. Therefore it is necessary to use a free tarsal graft, nasal cartilage, or buccal mucous membrane to line the flap.

Although we prefer a procedure in which upper lid donor material is advanced to fill the defect, the procedure can be used to fill defects greater than one half the length of the lid.

General anesthesia is preferred for this extensive dissection. A large central defect in the lower lid should be trimmed to a pentagonal shape (Plate 7-9, *A*). Beginning at the lateral canthus, an incision is made superiorly and temporally. The inferior crus of the lateral canthal tendon is lysed at its insertion to the lateral orbital tubercle. A skin-muscle flap is dissected temporally.

If a defect greater than one half the length of the lid is to be filled, the incision is curved downward in front of the ear and a cheek rotation flap created.

The temporal flap is advanced, and the marginal wound is closed with the three-suture technique. The raw edge of the flap is lined if necessary. The temporal wound is closed with interrupted 6-0 silk sutures (Plate 7-9, *B*). The lateral canthus is closed with a vertical mattress suture.

A light dressing is applied. Superficial sutures are removed after 4 days and the lid margin and mattress sutures 3 days later.

Plate 7-9

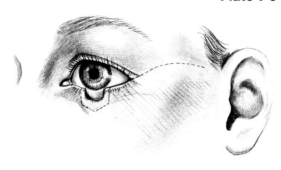

A, Large central defect with outline
of pentagonal incision and
temporal flap.

B, Flap advanced and sutured into
defect and then closed with
interrupted sutures.

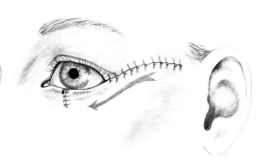

As a result of superficial traumatic, chemical, or thermal injury, the external layer of the lower lid may be contracted. The temporal transposition flap is particularly useful for the replacement of the skin and orbicularis layers of the lid, when the internal layers are viable. A free skin graft may be used in this area; however, if the defect extends beyond the lateral canthus and subcutaneous tissue is excised, a depression may result.

If general anesthesia is not used for this procedure, akinesia should be achieved with 2% lidocaine with 1:100,000 epinephrine.

A horizontal incision is made along the superior aspect of the fibrotic area, parallel to the lid margin. The skin and underlying tissue retracting the lid are dissected free and excised. The defect is trimmed to a workable contour (Plate 7-10, A).

A clever device for estimating the length and position of the flap is to hold a strip of gauze at the temporal end of the dissection and measure the length of the defect. With the temporal end of the gauze held in place, the material is rotated upward and used to ascertain the limits of the flap, which are outlined with a marking pencil.

The vertical transposition flap is incised with a knife blade and, beginning at its apex, dissected to include skin and enough subcutaneous tissue to include a vascular bed. If the length of this flap is greater than 2½ times its width, its transposition should be delayed (as previously described).

The base of the flap is sufficiently undermined to permit its easy transposition.

The donor bed is closed by extensive undermining of the adjacent wound edges and the use of 4-0 silk or nylon near-far, far-near sutures interspersed with interrupted 6-0 silk sutures. If the wound is wide enough, subcutaneous suturing with absorbable sutures may be necessary.

The surgeon sutures the flap into place with interrupted sutures of 6-0 silk, first orienting it into position with the extremities secured (Plate 7-10, B). Hemostasis should be achieved in the recipient area with moderate pressure rather than with cautery.

The area superior to the base of the flap is not sutured, because pressure might compromise the circulation in the flap. This area will eventually granulate.

A light Telfa dressing is applied. Superficial sutures are removed after 4 days and near-far, far-near sutures 3 days later. Adhesive strips are then applied for about 1 week to the donor site. Three weeks following the initial surgery the base of the flap may be released and that area modified.

The flap tends to be thickened for several weeks until the edema subsides. Further modification should be performed 6 months later.

Plate 7-10

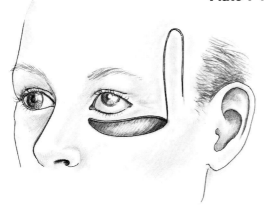

A, Temporal transposition flaps. Horizontal incision made through skin and subcutaneous tissue and subsequent dissection to release lower lid. Temporal flap dissected. Note presence of subcutaneous tissue.

B, Temporal flap transposed and sutured into defect. Donor site closed with near-far, far-near sutures.

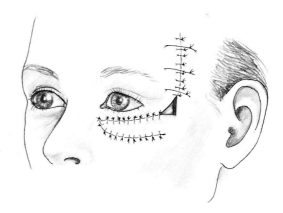

As has been mentioned, it is our opinion that the procedure of choice in the repair of large defects of the upper lid is the use of a pedicle bridge flap from the ipsilateral lower lid. However, in those cases in which there has also been substantial loss of lower lid tissue making that lid unsuited as a donor site, the use of transposed pedicle flaps is indicated. Since these flaps replace the full thickness of the lid, it is necessary to line them with mucous membrane as a protection for the globe. Although nasal cartilage is suitable for this purpose, it is also possible to line the pedicle flaps with buccal mucous membrane before its transposition.

This is an especially useful technique when the lid defect, although of full thickness, does not involve the margin of the lid with its tarsal plate. Here a mucous membrane lining is required, but the rigidity of nasal cartilage is not necessary.

If the procedure is not performed under general anesthesia, adequate akinesia should be achieved with 2% lidocaine with 1:100,000 epinephrine.

A methylene blue marking pencil is used to outline the area of the donor flap after a gauze strip has been used as a measuring device to estimate the size and location of the flap (Plate 7-11, A).

The transposition flap is incised and dissected to a depth that will ensure the presence of a good vascular bed. The flap is dissected from its apex toward the base.

The mucous membrane graft is then obtained. With the lower lip everted on an appropriate clamp or two towel hooks, the inside of the lip is injected with 1% lidocaine with 1:100,000 epinephrine, regardless of the type of anesthesia used.

A Castroviejo mucotome is then used to obtain a graft that is 0.5 mm thick (Plate 7-11, B). The clamp is removed from the lip and wet gauze is placed over the wound.

The mucous membrane is immediately transferred to a piece of Gelfilm. The graft is stapled to it with a small stapling device, with its smooth side toward the Gelfilm. The Gelfilm with the attached mucous membrane is trimmed to two thirds the length of the transposition flap and to an equal width.

The graft stapled to the Gelfilm is then sutured with 4-0 chromic sutures to the subcutaneous part of the transposition flap, with the raw surface of the mucous membrane toward the underside of the flap. The flap is replaced in its bed and sutured with 6-0 silk sutures to allow for longitudinal vascularization and adherence of the graft (Plate 7-11, C). A light dressing is applied. The 6-0 silk sutures are removed after 4 days.

Plate 7-11

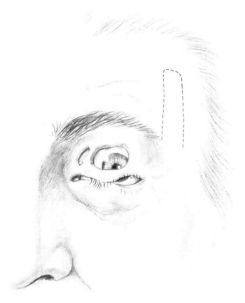

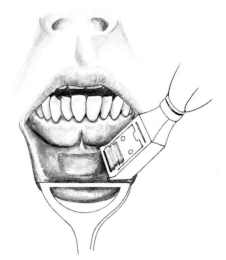

A, Large fistulizing defect of upper lid with outline of delayed pedicle flap.

B, Castroviejo mucotome used to obtain donor mucous membrane.

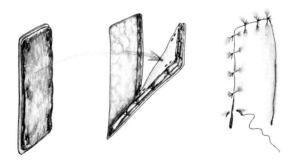

C, Mucous membrane stapled to Gelfilm and sutured to underside of flap. Flap resutured into original position.

After 30 days, the second stage of the procedure is performed. The recipient area is trimmed to the approximate size of the transposition flap it is to receive. A knife is used to incise the flap, and blunt dissection is used to reach the level of the mucous membrane. The flap is raised and the Gelfilm carefully removed (Plate 7-11, *D*).

At that time the base of the flap is sufficiently dissected to allow for easy transposition. The donor site is closed, as has been previously described, with undermining and the use of near-far, far-near sutures.

The flap is closed in layers. The mucous membrane is sutured with 6-0 chromic suture to the remaining conjunctiva. The orbicularis layer, which is sutured to the subcutaneous layer of the flap, is closed with 5-0 chromic suture. The skin is closed with interrupted 6-0 silk sutures. Once again, the triangle at the base of the flap is allowed to granulate (Plate 7-11, *E*). A marginal suture is placed from the lower lid margin and anchored to the brow.

A light gauze dressing is applied. The superficial sutures are removed after 5 days. The near-far, far-near sutures and the marginal suture are removed after 1 week. Three weeks following the transposition, the base of the flap can be lysed and the area modified.

The flap tends to remain edematous for several weeks. Occasionally, a procedure is needed to thin the flap. Scar revision and dermabrasion, if needed, can be performed several months after surgery.

Plate 7·11, cont'd

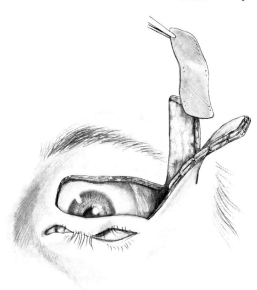

D, Upper lid fistulas excised. Temporal flap raised and Gelfilm removed.

E, Flap transposed and sutured into position. Marginal lid suture placed. Donor site closed.

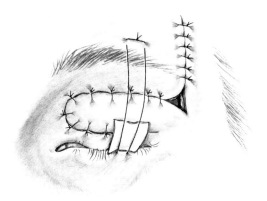

The need for reconstruction of the lateral canthus is generally secondary to lesions that involve the substance of both the upper and lower lids at the lateral canthal angle. Basal cell carcinoma, a common cause of defects in this area, responds poorly to other forms of treatment, and complete surgical excision is the only sure form of therapy. When recurrences do occur, they probably result from incomplete incision due to faulty technique. The surgeon is often reluctant to perform the excision necessary for absolute certainty of eradication because of apprehension at the thought of having to perform a reconstructive procedure in this difficult-to-handle area. Therefore we recommend that lesions in this area be excised widely and deeply. Frozen sections should be made if facilities are available: marginal specimens are sent for permanent section.

The globe should be adequately protected during surgery with a contact shell. A local anesthetic (2% lidocaine with 1:100,000 epinephrine) is injected following delineation of the lines of incision with a marking pencil (Plate 7-12, *A*).

The initial incisions through the lid are perpendicular to the lid margin. These are carried vertically to the fornices and then turned temporally to widely circumscribe the lesion. The canthus is rotated outward so that the depth of the excision can be ascertained (Plate 7-12, *B*). Lesions in this area will often require excision down to periosteum. If there is periosteal involvement, this tissue also must be excised.

The specimen should then be completely removed and properly oriented and labeled on a piece of Telfa or other suitable background. The margins of the lesion are examined by the pathologist as separate specimens, including the base of the tissue. Having been reasonably assured following frozen section examination that the margins are clear, the surgeon can proceed to reconstruct the area.

The upper lid is everted and stabilized with a traction suture or an appropriate lid clamp or both. An incision is made with a razor blade knife 3 mm from the lid margin through the conjunctiva and tarsus wide enough to fill the lateral defect.

The medial end of this incision is extended high into the fornix. With a Westcott scissors the tarsoconjunctival flap is dissected in a plane between Müller's fibers and the levator aponeurosis. When the dissection has been carried sufficiently high into the fornix so that the flap can be easily transposed without causing an arching of the upper lid, the lateral transposition is made. The inferior edge of the flap is sutured to the remaining conjunctiva of the lower lid with 5-0 chromic catgut suture. The temporal edge of the lower lid is grooved, and a 6-0 mattress suture is passed from inside the lid through the medial aspect of the flap to be withdrawn on the skin surface (Plate 7-12, *C*). The overlying skin of the lateral canthus is undermined, and sliding advancement flaps are prepared.

Plate 7-12

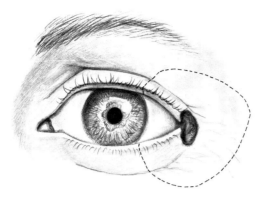

A, Malignant lesion of lateral canthus with outline of area to be excised.

B, Full-thickness incision down to conjunctiva.

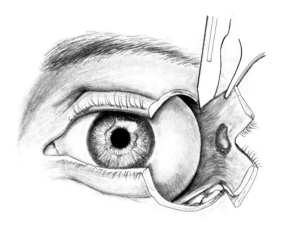

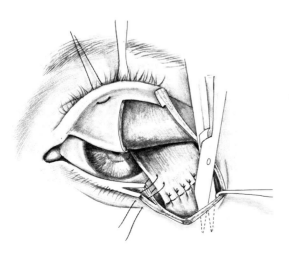

C, Tarsoconjunctival flap transposed from upper lid and sutured into defect. Note mattress suture through intramarginal groove. Adjacent skin being undermined.

A trapdoor flap is now made from periosteum at the lateral canthus. If periosteum has been taken, holes can be drilled into bone for this purpose. A 6-0 mattress suture is placed from this flap through a groove slot that is created in the medial aspect of the upper lid. The lower lid mattress suture is then tied over a cotton bolster (Plate 7-12, *D*).

The initial suture through the new canthal tendon is also tied over a cotton bolster, and more absorbable sutures are placed to secure this to the flap. The sliding skin flaps are then advanced at the lateral canthus (Plate 7-12, *E*). The surgeon closes the skin layer with interrupted 6-0 silk sutures, trimming the skin flap where necessary (Plate 7-12, *F*).

A light dressing is applied and changed daily for several days. The mattress sutures are removed after 1 week.

Following a 4- to 6-week period, the tarsorrhaphy is severed and the wound edges trimmed and sutured at the new mucocutaneous junction with 6-0 absorbable sutures, which can be removed after 1 week.

Plate 7-12, cont'd

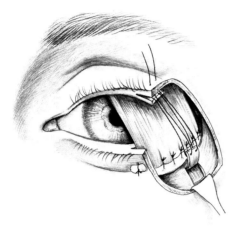

D, Periosteal hinged flap being created and sutured to upper lid to re-create lateral canthal tendon.

E, New lateral canthal tendon sutured in place. Skin flap advanced.

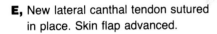
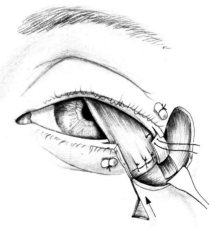

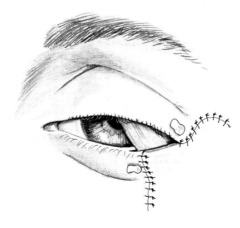

F, Skin closure effected with interrupted 6-0 silk suture.

Reconstruction of the medial canthus, like repair at the lateral canthus, follows the excision of malignancies in this area.

The excision of lesions in the medial canthus requires reconstructive techniques that generally are more involved than those at the lateral canthus. The anatomy of this area is more complex, with the presence of the medial canthal tendon and the lacrimal system: puncti, canaliculi, and tear sac. If the complete excision of the lesion requires removal of these elements of the lacrimal system, then not only must the anatomic configuration of the lids and medial canthal angle be reconstituted, but the lacrimal drainage system must also be recreated.

Generally, at the time of surgery the area that is to be excised is outlined with a methylene blue marking pencil (Plate 7-13, A). The initial perpendicular incisions through the lid margins are made through an area in which the architecture of the meibomian orifices is intact. Distortion and obliteration of these orifices are evidence of tissue involvement in this area.

The incisions are extended to the fornices and then turned horizontally to widely circumscribe the mass. The angular vessels are usually encountered at the canthal angle, and hemostasis is achieved. At this point the surgeon determines by visual examination or frozen section if the lacrimal structures need to be excised. If this is needed, the dissection is extended down to periosteum (Plate 7-13, B). This en bloc specimen and the previously mentioned peripheral sections are submitted to the pathology department.

For the surgeon who performs this operation infrequently, closure of most canthal defects is probably best achieved by awaiting gradual granulation of the area. This technique enables the surgeon to concentrate on the complete eradication of the lesion without the worry of a somewhat complicated reconstructive technique.

After the excision has been completed, the lids are closed and held together with interrupted 6-0 silk sutures tied over a cotton pledget (Plate 7-13, C). This area is packed with a petrolatum dressing and then covered with a loose gauze dressing. The loose dressing is changed daily, with great care not to disrupt the new granulating tissue. The petrolatum dressing is removed and changed every 3 to 4 days. After complete granulation has occurred, the medial canthal angle may need to be surgically modified. If epiphora results, the lacrimal drainage can be reconstituted with the use of a curved polyethylene tube inserted from the canthus into the nasolacrimal duct. This relatively simple technique offers excellent results, with no need to resort to a reconstructive technique.

Plate 7-13

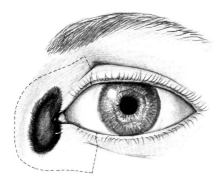

A, Large medial canthal lesion involving lacriminal excretory system. Area to be excised outlined.

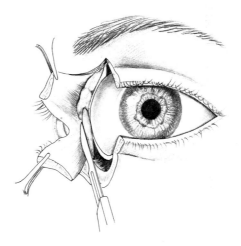

B, Dissection extended down to expose full extent of lesion.

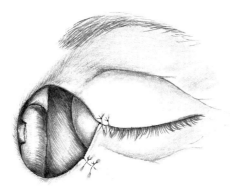

C, Lids closed and sutured together.

For the more experienced surgeon, the technique we prefer is a tarsoconjunctival graft taken from the upper lid.

The upper lid is everted and reflected temporally. A razor blade knife is used to incise the conjunctiva and tarsus 2 to 3 mm from the lid margin (Plate 7-14, *A*). The incision is extended temporally to create a flap about the size of the defect to be filled. The dissection is made sufficiently high into the cul-de-sac, between the tarsus and the retractors of the upper lid (levator aponeurosis and Müller's muscle), to allow its medial transposition.

The tarsoconjunctival flap is then brought down into position in the lower fornix and sutured to what remains of the conjunctiva with absorbable 6-0 sutures. The stump of the medial canthal tendon, if it remains, is sutured to the tarsoconjunctival graft with 5-0 nylon sutures (Plate 7-14, *B*). If the medial canthal tendon stump is not present, then the graft is sutured with 5-0 (35 gauge) stainless steel wire to the anterior lacrimal crest after this has been drilled with several holes.

Next, the surgeon prepares the lower lid to receive the tarsoconjunctival graft by creating a groove in it, into which interdigitates the inferolateral aspect of the graft (Plate 7-14, *C*). A 6-0 silk mattress suture is used, woven from the inside out to hold this area in position.

Plate 7-14

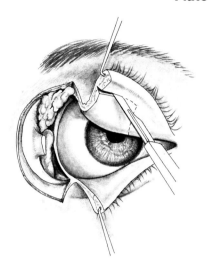

A, Preparation of tarsoconjunctival flap. Note 2 to 3 mm area of lid margin preserved.

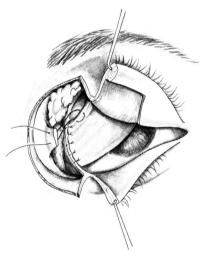

B, Flap transposed and sutured into position. Stump of medial canthal tendon sutured to tarsal flap.

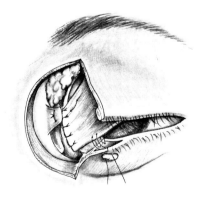

C, Medial canthal tendon recreated. Graft being sutured into lower lid groove.

The closure of the overlying wound is best achieved by the use of a free full-thickness skin graft. There is no readily available skin for the creation of advancement flaps in the medial canthal area; therefore full-thickness skin preferably is taken from the contralateral upper lid, or a retroauricular graft may be used as a second choice, since this skin is an excellent match in the lid area.

The skin graft is cut to the shape of the defect (Plate 7-14, D) and sutured into place with interrupted 6-0 silk sutures. The suture ends are left about 1½ inches long. The graft is then perforated with multiple incisions to prevent fluid accumulation beneath it.

The suture ends, which have been left long, are tied over a cotton or synthetic bolster (Telfa), which also helps prevent fluid accumulation beneath the graft (Plate 7-14, E). A Frost suture is generally placed and tied over pledgets to keep the lid in position for approximately 4 to 5 days. The bolster is removed after 3 days and the silk suture after 5 to 6 days. With the packing secured over the graft, a light dressing is applied.

The surgeon must be careful to begin the initial incision 2 to 3 mm from the lid margin or an entropion may result, which may require surgical correction. If the tarsoconjunctival graft is stretched to reach the recipient area and not dissected high enough into the cul-de-sac, arching of the lid will result. "Rounding" of the medial canthal angle is a possibility and may need to be modified later with a medial canthoplasty. Fluid accumulation beneath the skin graft may result in sloughing of the graft. Care must be taken to incise the graft and to apply gentle pressure with a nonadhesive dressing.

Plate 7-14, cont'd

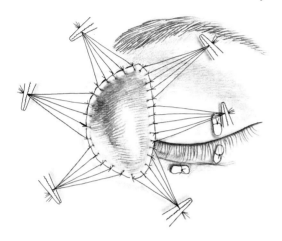

D, Free skin graft placed over defect.

E, Bolster tied over graft with suture ends.

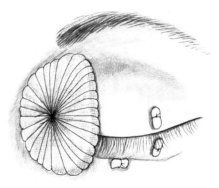

CHAPTER 8

ENTROPION REPAIR

Entropion, the inward rotation of the lid margin, can from a practical surgical standpoint be divided into two types: cicatricial and noncicatricial. In the involutional (noncicatricial) type of entropion, there is generally a laxity in the lid tissues, which causes the pretarsal orbicularis to loosen its attachment to the underlying tarsal fascia. The result is an overriding of the pretarsal orbicularis by the preseptal orbicularis and a subsequent inward turning of the lid margin.

Generally, if the degree of entropion is not too severe, correction can be achieved with a relatively simple and popular procedure, in which a triangular piece of tissue is resected and sutured closed, causing the lid margin to evert.

BASE-DOWN-TRIANGLE TARSAL RESECTION (Plate 8-1)

After suitable lid akinesia has been achieved with 2% lidocaine with 1:100,000 epinephrine, a chalazion clamp is placed at about two thirds the distance from the medial to the lateral canthus (Plate 8-1, A). The clamp should be sufficiently large to expose the full dimension of the tarsus. Using a razor blade knife, the surgeon outlines a triangle, with its base at the lower tarsal margin and its apex about 2 mm from the lid margin. The triangle should be incised through the conjunctiva and down to the tarsus (Plate 8-1, B). To be effective, the base of the triangle must be from 7 to 10 mm in length. The triangle is excised with the razor blade knife, with dissection extended down to the pretarsal orbicularis.

Following the incision of this tarsoconjunctival base-down triangle, three to four 5-0 or 6-0 chromic catgut sutures should be placed across the defect so that when tied the knots will be buried within the wound (Plate 8-1, C).

Before the sutures are tied, the chalazion clamp should be loosened and the sutures tied from the base outward (Plate 8-1, D). The chalazion clamp is then removed; a small elevation of the lid margin is usually present, which disappears within several weeks (Plate 8-1, E). The sutures are left to be absorbed but they could be removed after 7 to 8 days if necessary.

Plate 8-1

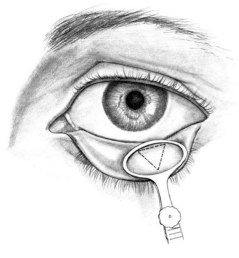

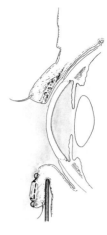

A, Chalazion clamp placed on lower lid with area to be resected outlined.

B, Sagittal section to show depth of incision.

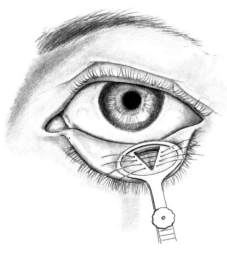

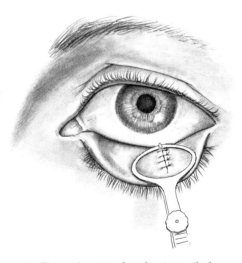

C, Sutures placed across surgical defect in tarsus.

D, Clamp loosened and sutures tied.

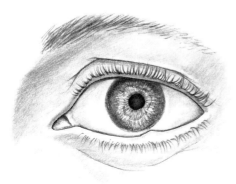

E, Lid position at end of procedure. Note small elevation of lid margin.

When the amount of entropion is somewhat greater or when the previous procedure has proved inadequate to correct the condition, our next procedure of choice is the orbicularis transplant. In this procedure a strip of orbicularis is dissected free through a blepharoplasty incision. The temporal end of the strip is transposed and attached to the periosteum of the inferior orbital rim, thus physically extra-rotating the lid margin and at the same time causing a scarring between the pretarsal orbicularis, the preseptal orbicularis, and the underlying tissue.

Once again the procedure is begun by placing a contact shell on the globe. A methylene blue marking pencil is used to mark a line about 2 to 3 mm below the lash line, extending from just below the punctum to the temporal smile crease (Plate 8-2, *A*). The area is then infiltrated with 2% lidocaine with 1:100,000 epinephrine, in this case for lid akinesia and hydraulic dissection. A razor blade knife is then used to incise along the demarcated line. A lid plate can be used for support during this step (Plate 8-2, *B*).

The skin overlying the lower lid is dissected free from the orbicularis muscle with a Westcott scissors and forceps. The dissection is carried down to the inferior orbital rim (Plate 8-2, *C*).

Plate 8-2

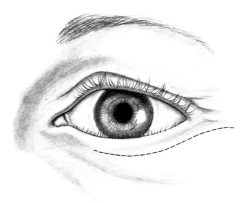

A, Outline of subciliary incision to be made.

B, Lid plate in place and skin incision being made.

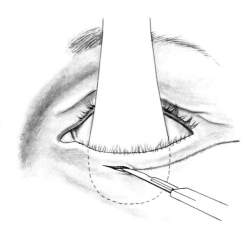

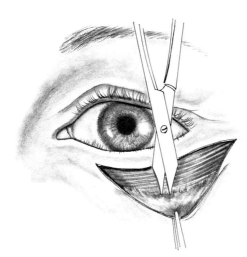

C, Skin dissected free from underlying orbicularis.

About 3 mm below the lash line, the orbicularis is incised parallel to the initial skin incision from its medial aspect to its temporal extremity. A strip of orbicularis muscle, which should be at least 7 to 10 mm wide to include the pretarsal and preseptal portions, is then prepared. A muscle hook is useful in grasping the muscle while the underlying fascia is dissected free (Plate 8-2, *D* and *E*).

At the temporal extremity of the dissection, the orbicularis strip is cut free (Plate 8-2, *F*). At this point the surgeon must decide if orbital fat should be excised. If so, then after the septum has been opened with the spreading action of a hemostat or blunt scissors, the fat that is easily prolapsable is gently grasped with minimal traction and clamped. The fat is excised (Plate 8-2, *G*) and careful hemostasis achieved with cautery before the fat is released. The septum can be closed with interrupted absorbable sutures; most recently we have not been doing so.

Plate 8-2, cont'd

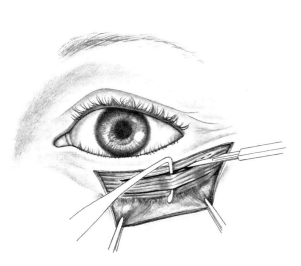

D, Strip of orbicularis (10 mm wide) dissected free.

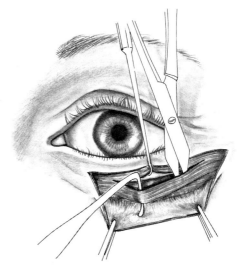

E, Orbicularis dissected free from underlying tissue.

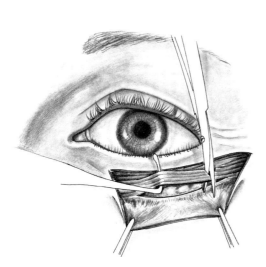

F, Temporal extremity of orbicularis strip released.

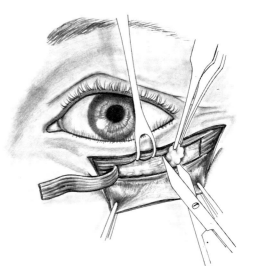

G, Excision of prolapsing orbital fat.

The temporal extremity of the strip is then grasped with a hemostat. On the temporal aspect of the inferior orbital rim, a scissors is used to dissect down to periosteum, although formerly this dissection was extended only to septum (Plate 8-2, *H*).

A doubled-armed 4-0 absorbable suture is passed through the periosteum two times and passed through the temporal aspect of the orbicularis band (Plate 8-2, *I*).

The tension of the band is adjusted as it is tied down to the periosteum. Excessive traction will cause deformity of the lid margin in the opposite direction. Two more 4-0 absorbable sutures are placed to secure the strip in position (Plate 8-2, *J*).

The overlying skin is then placed over the lid margin and excessive skin excised as in a lower lid blepharoplasty. Interrupted or continuous 6-0 or 7-0 silk sutures are placed to close the incision (Plate 8-2, *K*). A light dressing is applied. Sutures are removed after 4 to 5 days.

Plate 8-2, cont'd

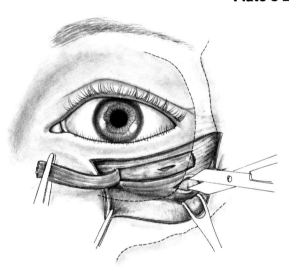

H, Dissection extended to level of periosteum of inferior orbital rim.

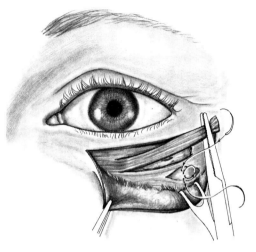

I, Temporal extremity of orbicularis band ready to be sutured to periosteum.

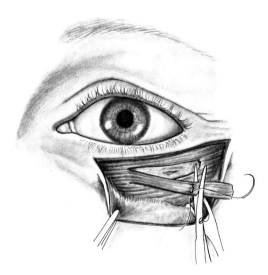

J, Tension of band adjusted and excess tissue excised.

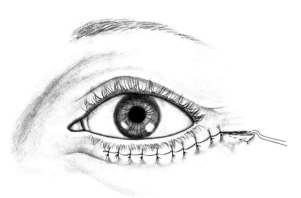

K, Redundant skin to be excised and skin layer closed.

TARSAL WEDGE

(Plate 8-3)

The tarsal wedge procedure is successful in cases of cicatricial entropion of the upper lid in which there is a minimal amount of lid tissue and in which the contralateral upper lid offers an adequate free tarsal graft. For example, this procedure is particularly well suited to correct an inward turning of the central portion of the left upper lid.

The contralateral upper lid is first everted on an Erhardt or other suitable lid clamp just above the lower tarsal border, and a triangular strip of tarsus, 2 mm at its base, is marked and incised (Plate 8-3, *A*). The triangular donor graft is excised with a razor blade knife and carefully handled before its repositioning (Plate 8-3, *B*). In this case the donor site is not sutured but allowed to freely granulate.

With the involved lid in an everted position and secured with twin forceps, the area of the inwardly rotated lid is then incised about 2 mm from the lid margin on the tarsal surface (Plate 8-3, *C*). This incision should be made at a 45-degree angle to the plane of the tarsus. The base of the incision then acts as a hinge to extrarotate the lid (Plate 8-3, *D*) and provide a site for placement of the donor graft.

Plate 8-3

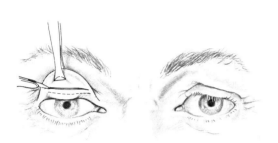

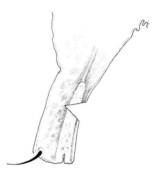

A, Entropion of left upper lid. Right upper lid everted and donor graft site marked and incised.

B, Sagittal view of upper lid to show site of donor graft.

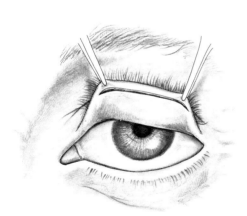

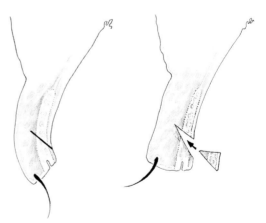

C, Incision made into tarsus of entropic lid.

D, Sagittal view demonstrating direction of incision through entropic lid and donor graft to be placed therein.

TARSAL WEDGE—cont'd

Using two 6-0 silk double-armed sutures that are placed at the triangular apices on either end of the graft, the surgeon places the tarsal graft into the recipient bed. The sutures are passed through the full thickness of the lid but do not exit the conjunctival surface of the lid (Plate 8-3, *E*).

The wedge is sutured into place with interrupted absorbable sutures (Plate 8-3, *F*). The position of the donor graft should be such that the hinged outer aspect of the lid extra-rotates and assumes a normal position (Plate 8-3, *G*).

Plate 8-3, cont'd

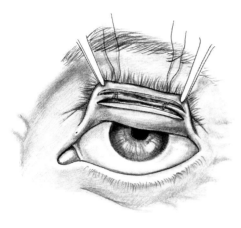

E, Double-armed suture through apex of graft and pulled full thickness through upper lid.

F, Tarsal graft put in place with interrupted sutures.

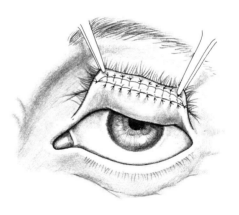

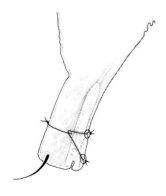

G, Sagittal view of wedge sutured into position.

For a more severe degree of cicatrization of the upper lid or in those cases in which a previous attempt at correction has failed, the procedure that we prefer is the through-and-through fracturing of the tarsus combined with the external rotation of the entire lid margin. Often, not only do these cases involve the scarring of the inside layer of the lid, but also, as in alkali burns, there is complete shrinkage of all of the layers of the lid. Therefore a procedure that affects only internal or external layers of that lid would not be sufficient for correction.

After the placement of a protective contact shell and following adequate local infiltration of anesthetic, if general anesthesia is not used, the inwardly rotated lid is grasped on its external surface and outwardly rotated. About 4 mm above the lash line a methylene blue marking pencil is used to designate the line of incision from the medial to the temporal aspect of the lid beyond the area of lid malposition (Plate 8-4, *A*).

A razor blade knife is then used to incise along the line down through the skin and into the orbicularis (Plate 8-4, *B*). A full-thickness penetration is not sought because of the possibility of angling the incision and of damaging the marginal arterial arcade, which is present within 3 mm of the lid margin.

Instead the lid is everted, and with the lid margin in view an incision at a similar distance is made through the tarsus and the conjunctiva (Plate 8-4, *C*).

Plate 8-4

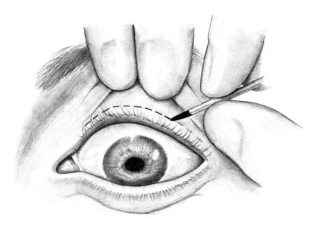

A, Inverted lid margin extra-rotated and line of incision marked.

B, Horizontal incision made through skin and orbicularis.

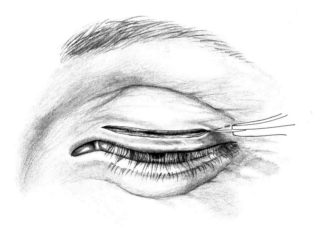

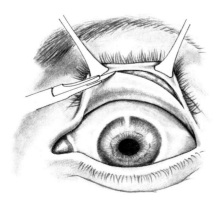

C, Upper lid everted and tarsus incised opposite skin incision.

With the lid in the normal position, a Westcott scissors is used to complete the transverse blepharotomy incision (Plate 8-4, *D*).

The lid margin having been freed, a 4-0 double-armed suture is passed centrally from the conjunctival side of the lid tissue through the tarsus and withdrawn from the middle lamella of the upper aspect of the wound (Plate 8-4, *E*). This double-armed suture is then passed through the lid margin bridge and withdrawn just above the lash line (Plate 8-4, *F*).

Plate 8-4, cont'd

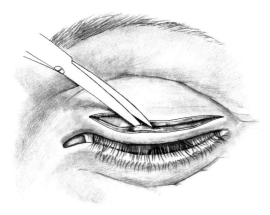

D, Scissors used to join two incisions.

E, Double-armed silk suture placed from conjunctival level outward.

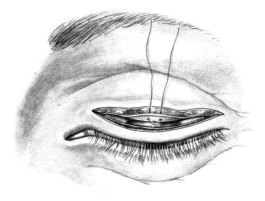

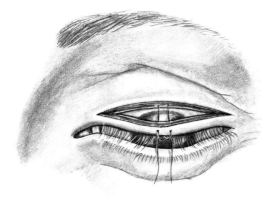

F, Suture brought through lid margin above lash line.

The inwardly turned upper lid margin has now been transversely incised and the marginal strip of lid externally rotated and secured into its new position (Plate 8-4, *G*).

Approximately four to five of these 4-0 double-armed sutures are placed (Plate 8-4, *H*). These are tied sufficiently tight to ensure a slight overcorrection of the lid margin. These sutures can be tied over cotton bolsters.

The upper skin edge is closed with interrupted 6-0 silk sutures, and a light dressing is applied. These are removed after 4 days and the mattress sutures after 1 week.

Plate 8-4, cont'd

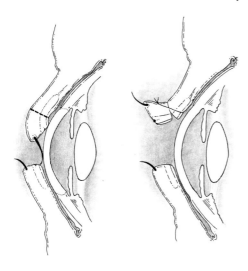

G, Sagittal view demonstrating entropic upper lid and placement of initial suture.

H, Lid in final position with several double-armed sutures in place and skin closed.

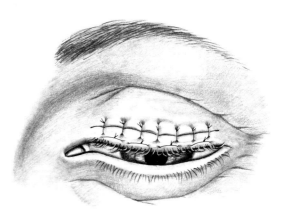

CHAPTER 9

ECTROPION REPAIR

For surgical purposes we generally divide ectropion, the outward turning of the lid margin, into two types: cicatricial and noncicatricial. The noncicatricial type generally results from an involutional process in which there is a gradual laxity in the tissues of the lower lid combined with a laxity of the supporting structures, the medial and lateral canthal tendons, of that lid. Because of this laxity, there is a subsequent increase in the horizontal length of the lid. As time passes, a cicatrization of the lid tissues is produced within the lid, and thus a cicatricial component is added to the process. In a cicatricial ectropion there is a contracture of the anterior tissues of the lid, which causes an outward turning of the lid margin. As time passes, this produces a horizontal lengthening of the lid, a factor that must be taken into account when surgical correction of this entity is undertaken.

The surgical repair of noncicatricial ectropion is generally performed by correcting the entity that produces the deformity, that is, the horizontal lengthening and laxity of the lid. To fully ascertain the degree of horizontal laxity, it is generally necessary to free the vertically shortened and fibrosed external layers of the lid from the inner lamellae. After these fibrotic tissues, the cicatricial element of the ectropion, have been separated from the remainder of the lid, one can better ascertain the true degree of laxity that is present.

In those cases in which the cicatricial component produces a shortage of external tissue, it is necessary to replace this tissue with a free skin graft or to employ one of the other procedures that have been previously described.

For the correction of an involutional ectropion with a lateral or complete eversion of the lid margin, we generally perform a full-thickness horizontal shortening of the lid under a blepharoplasty-type skin flap.

After a protective contact shell has been placed over the globe, a methylene blue marking pencil is used to designate an area for a subciliary incision about 3 mm below the lash line and extending from just below the punctum to the temporal smile fold at the lateral canthus (Plate 9-1, A). The lid is then anesthetized with 2% lidocaine with 1:100,000 epinephrine to provide lid akinesia and hydraulic dissection.

After the skin is incised along the demarcated area with a razor blade knife, the skin is separated from the underlying orbicularis down to the level of the inferior orbital rim. The dissection is slowly and carefully performed so as not to macerate the orbicularis fibers. The hydraulic dissection achieved with the local injection of anesthetic usually facilitates this maneuver, although usually students find this part of the procedure difficult to master. With the skin adequately dissected from the orbicularis, the lid is now freely movable and the full degree of laxity is demonstrable (Plate 9-1, B).

About one third the distance from the lateral canthus, a full-thickness incision is made through the lid margin to about 2 mm below the tarsus. The incision then turns medially to form half of a pentagon. The lateral aspect of the lid is overlapped by the remainder of the lid, and the amount of tissue that needs to be excised is ascertained. The pentagonal wedge is then completed in the desired area. The second incision should be made parallel to the first so that lid closure results in a uniform lid margin with no notching of the lid.

The lid margin is closed by the three-suture technique, with the tarsal layer closed in this case to include overlying orbicularis. Absorbable 5-0 sutures are used for the closure (Plate 9-1, C).

The skin flap is drawn up and gently pulled laterally; any redundant skin is excised (Plate 9-1, D). If the cicatricial component has been extensive, the external layer of the lid may have to be replaced. The incision is then closed with interrupted or continuous 6-0 silk sutures (Plate 9-1, E).

A light dressing is applied to the wound. This is generally removed on the final postoperative day. The skin sutures are removed after 4 days and the marginal sutures 3 days later.

Plate 9-1

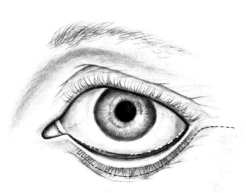

A, Subciliary incision outlined. Note temporal extension into smile fold.

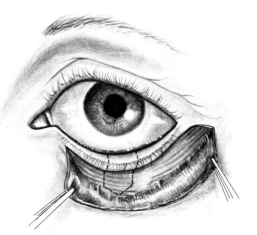

B, Skin dissected free from orbicularis and fibrotic tissue; pentagon-shaped excision outlined.

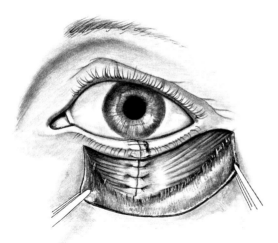

C, Lid horizontally shortened and closed with three-suture technique.

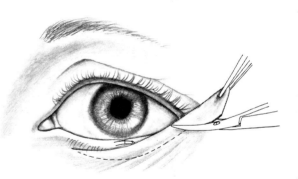

D, Redundant skin excised.

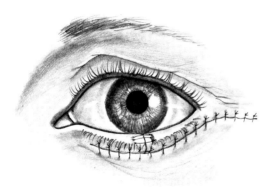

E, Closure with interrupted sutures.

When the ectropion involves the medial aspect of the lid, especially in those cases in which there is a frank punctal eversion resulting from horizontal lid laxity rather than a more distinct weakness of the medial canthal tendon, the procedure that we prefer is the lazy-T correction. In this procedure a V-shaped wedge is excised from the lid to correct the horizontal lengthening that may be present, while at the same time a horizontal incision through the conjunctiva and tarsus is used to correct the eversion of the lid (Plate 9-2, *A*). Although other techniques such as internal cautery of the lid and a horizontal excision of tarsoconjunctival tissue used alone have been advocated, we have found these to be fraught with complications (the former) or insufficient to correct the underlying pathophysiology of the defect (the latter).

For the lazy-T procedure we usually prefer general anesthesia, because this avoids distortion of the lid anatomy caused by local infiltration of anesthetic solution. However, if local anesthesia is used, the surgeon should allow about 15 minutes to elapse after injection to permit the solution to dissipate in the tissues.

After the placement of a contact shell over the globe, a forceps is used to evert the lower lid. It may also be helpful to support the lid with a lid plate during the first part of the procedure. A probe is then inserted into the canaliculus to locate its horizontal level in the lid. Approximately 7 mm below the punctum an incision is made with a razor blade knife through conjunctiva and tarsus. The incision should be about 1 to 1½ cm in length, with the medial aspect of the incision extending slightly beyond the punctum (Plate 9-2, *B*).

Plate 9-2

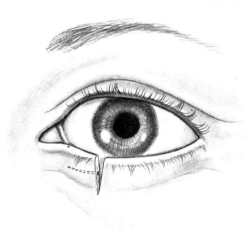

A, Combined horizontal and vertical
shortening to produce lazy T.

B, Initial incision through conjunctiva
and tarsus.

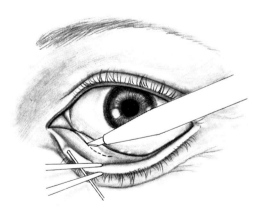

A scissors is then used to undermine the inferior edge of the wound. This undermining should extend for about 3 to 5 mm (Plate 9-2, *C* and *D*). With sufficient undermining, the inferior aspect of the incision can overlap the superior portion of the wound. It is useful to employ two forceps, each grasping an alternate end of the wound and thus facilitating the overlapping (Plate 9-2, *E* and *F*).

The inferior wound edge is gently dissected, and the correct lid position is determined. The entire area that has been undermined is excised so that the lid will be held in the position into which it is sutured (Plate 9-2, *G*).

Plate 9-2, cont'd

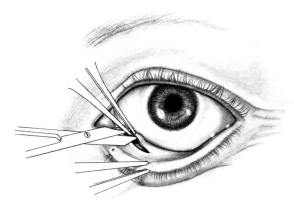

C, Inferior border of incision undermined.

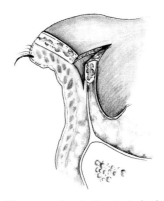

D, Cross section to illustrate incision.

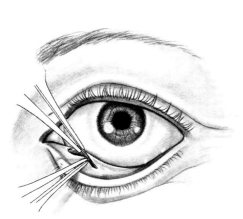

E, Inferior aspect of wound overlapped.

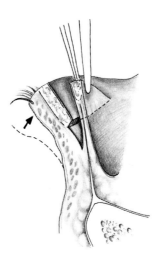

F, Cross section to illustrate overlapping.

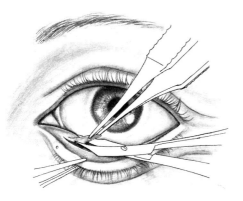

G, Excess tissue resected.

The horizontal lid laxity is then corrected by making a full-thickness vertical incision of the lid 3 mm lateral to the punctum down to the lower fornix (Plate 9-2, *H*). With the surgeon using the double-armed forceps technique, the two edges of the incision are overlapped and the area to be excised is determined (Plate 9-2, *I* and *J*). The resection is sufficient to correct the horizontal laxity and place the lid in correct apposition with the globe. The resection takes a triangular wedge shape in the lid, which can be closed by the three-suture technique previously described (Plate 9-2, *K*).

For closure of the horizontal tarsoconjunctival incision, we prefer 7-0 chromic catgut sutures. These are placed in an interrupted fashion and the knots pulled into the conjunctiva as much as possible. These generally cause no irritation.

With this part of the procedure completed, the lid is closed. A light dressing is applied. Superficial sutures are removed after 4 days and marginal sutures 3 days later.

Plate 9-2, cont'd

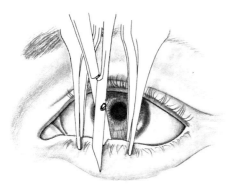

H, Full-thickness incision through lid margin.

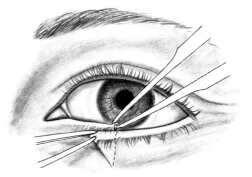

I, Lid margin overlapped and amount to be resected outlined.

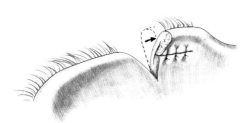

J, Inner aspect of lid to illustrate excessive lid tissue excised and tarsoconjunctival wound closed.

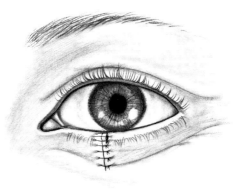

K, Closure of lid margin with three-suture technique.

CHAPTER 10

COSMETIC BLEPHAROPLASTY

Dermatochalasis refers to an excess of skin in the upper or lower lids commonly seen in the middle aged and elderly. Excessive skin overhanging the supratarsal crease can override the lashes and lid margin of the upper lid, while in the lower lid it can cause excessive bagging. This condition may be associated with allergy, infection, or metabolic disturbances. It should be differentiated from blepharochalasis, which is a hereditary condition affecting young people in which the lid tissues are atrophied, causing skin redundancy and herniation of fat through the orbital septum.

The procedures for correction of excessive lid skin are no longer reserved for those cases in which obstructive or fatigue symptoms occur (Plate 10-1, *A*). The current emphasis on youth has created an increasing need for the ophthalmologist to be familiar with these techniques.

Preoperatively a complete ophthalmologic evaluation of the patient should be performed. Photographic documentation is essential. Asymmetries of facial contour should be pointed out to the patient before surgery. A Schirmer test should be performed, since a mild overcorrection could cause a dry eye in a marginal case. Finally, systemic causes of lid swelling, such as renal or thyroid disorders, should be kept in mind.

The technique is generally performed with local anesthesia (2% lidocaine with 1:100,000 epinephrine). In younger patients with congenital dermatochalasia, general anesthesia can be used, but the lids should be injected in the same way to achieve hydraulic dissection and good hemostasis.

Following the placement of a contact shell to protect the globe, a methylene blue marking pencil is used to designate an area at or just (1 mm) below the supratarsal crease (Plate 10-1, *B*).

A fixation forceps with the lower blade placed along the demarcated line is used to grasp the redundant lid skin. The skin is elevated, and the superior margin of the skin to be excised is marked (Plate 10-1, *C*). The fixation forceps is moved from the temporal aspect of the lid to the medial aspect, and each section is marked accordingly (Plate 10-1, *D*).

Plate 10·1

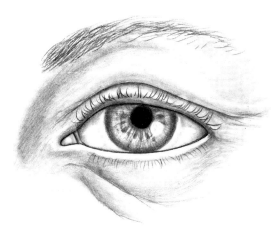

A, Excessive skin causing overhanging upper lid and bagging of lower lid.

B, Supratarsal crease marked.

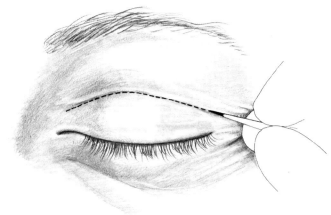

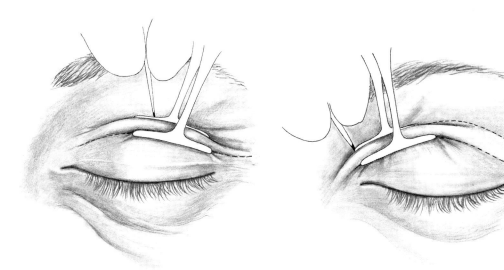

C, Fixation forceps used to determine amount of excessive skin to be removed.

D, Skin margins marked.

The redundant skin is ballooned away from the underlying orbicularis by the local anesthetic solution. Even with general anesthesia, this step will aid in dissection and facilitate postexcision hemostasis (Plate 10-1, *E*).

The upper lid is then held stretched with digital lateral pressure, and a Bard-Parker blade or preferably a razor blade fragment is used to incise the skin down to the orbicularis (Plate 10-1, *F*).

With the digital pressure maintained, the skin is excised from the lid with the blade or scissors. The assistant should continually control hemostasis with gentle pressure during the dissection so that the outline can be accurately followed (Plate 10-1, *G*). The excised skin is then placed in saline and refrigerated for 48 hours to be available for grafting in case of accidental overcorrection.

Plate 10-1, cont'd

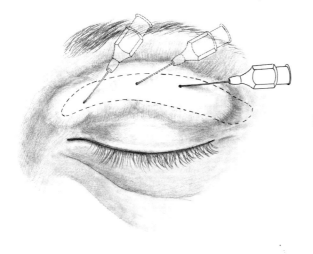

E, Local infiltration of anesthetic.

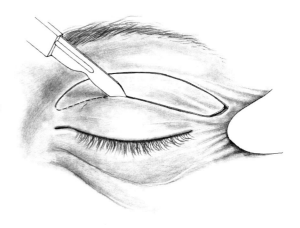

F, Incision of demarcated area down
to orbicularis.

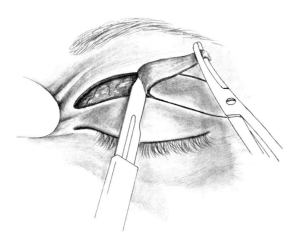

G, Skin resected while traction
digitally maintained.

Using a hemostat or blunt scissors, the surgeon carefully opens the orbicularis and orbital septum, avoiding insertion of any instrument too deeply into the lid, because this could damage the levator muscle or cause bleeding into the orbit (Plate 10-1, *H*).

With moderate pressure on the globe, preaponeurotic fat is prolapsed through the opening. Its capsule is gently opened with a scissors. The fat is never pulled, because this maneuver might damage vessels deep within the orbit. The fat is then clamped with a hemostat, and a knife blade is used to excise the fat above the clamp (Plate 10-1, *I*).

Before the hemostat is released, the fat is cauterized. This may not prevent bleeding behind the septum but will at least reduce the risk of local postoperative hematoma (Plate 10-1, *J*). Electrocautery of the orbicularis can be performed at this point, but we prefer mild pressure and vasoconstrictors. Fat can then be excised from as many areas as necessary in the upper lid. The septum is not sutured closed.

Plate 10-1, cont'd

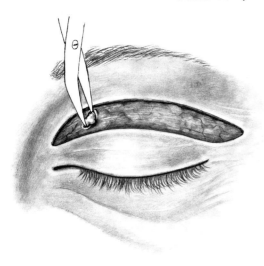

H, Blunt dissection through orbital septum performed and preaponeurotic fat prolapsed through opening.

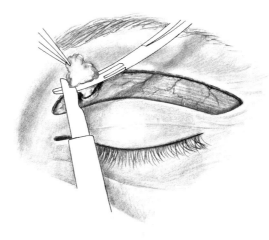

I, Prolapsing fat clamped and excised.

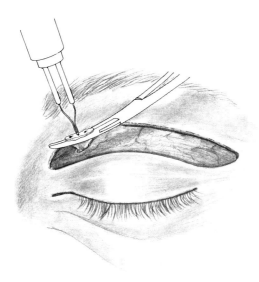

J, Fat carefully cauterized before being released.

The skin is then closed with fine 6-0 or 7-0 silk suture. Continuous suturing is also possible, but some experience is required to equalize suture tension with this technique. Subcuticular sutures can give an excellent cosmetic result, but we have found these difficult to remove, even if we leave a center loop in the lid.

Following the closure of the upper lid, the marking pencil is used to designate an area 2 to 3 mm below the lash line of the lower lid from just below the punctum to the temporal smile crease remaining at least 5 mm from the upper incision at this point to prevent webbing (Plate 10-1, K).

Following the injection of the local anesthetic, the blade is used to incise the previously demarcated area. The surgeon uses blunt scissors to separate the skin from the orbicularis, taking care not to macerate the underlying orbicularis, which may cause postoperative wadding and unsightly bulges in the lid. The dissection is carried to the level of the inferior orbital rim (Plate 10-1, L).

With care taken to release the surgical drape so that the cheek position will not be artificially elevated, the globe is gently depressed, and the amount of skin overlapping the incision is estimated. This skin is then excised in a double crescentic pattern so that a lateral lift can be given to the replaced skin (Plate 10-1, M). Excessive lower lid orbital fat is then excised as for the upper lid. The septum is not sutured.

The wound is closed with interrupted 6-0 silk sutures (Plate 10-1, N). At times it may be necessary to trim skin in the lateral canthus. Sutures are removed after 4 days.

No dressings are applied postoperatively. Application of cold compresses is begun in the recovery room to decrease swelling. The patients are advised to remain out of direct sunlight for several months.

A possible complication of lower lid blepharoplasty is ectropion resulting from lid flaccidity. This should be evaluated preoperatively and a horizontal shortening performed at the time of surgery. Cysts and suture tunnels that develop can be easily treated with excision or light cautery done as an office procedure.

Plate 10-1, cont'd

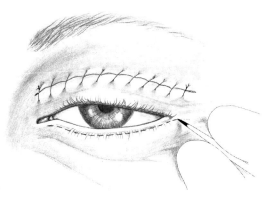

K, Skin on upper lid closed with 6-0 silk sutures and lower lid just below cilia marked.

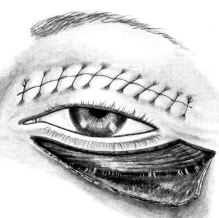

L, Subciliary incision made, carried to lateral smile crease, and then dissected free from orbicularis.

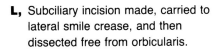

M, Excess skin excised as shown.

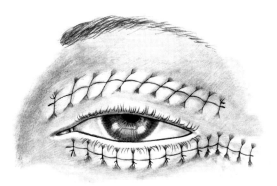

N, Skin closed with interrupted 6-0 silk sutures.

CHAPTER 11

LACRIMAL GLAND SURGERY

The lacrimal gland is located in the lacrimal fossa of the frontal bone under the superior temporal rim of the orbit. The gland is divided into two lobes, the orbital and palpebral lobes, by the lateral horn of the levator aponeurosis.

Reflex tear secretion is derived from the main lacrimal gland and its palpebral portion. The orbital portion of the gland has four to five ducts that empty above the border of the lateral tarsus. The 15 to 40 ducts of the palpebral portion empty into a common duct, which empties near the main ducts. Excision of the palpebral portion of the gland will most certainly destroy the ducts from the main gland. While the orbital portion of the gland is firmly supported by multiple ligaments in its fossa, the palpebral portion is not and may prolapse downward.

To begin this section with a warning to the surgeon would not be out of place. Palpebral lacrimal lobectomy should be performed only in carefully selected cases. When excessive tearing is an extremely irritating problem to the patient, and when all other means of care have been ruled out because of age or debilitation, then this procedure might be considered. In addition, success with this procedure is feasible in those cases in which lacrimal excretory surgery, with an in-place nasolacrimal tube, has been successfully performed and tearing still persists.

Surgery should be performed on one eye at a time, with a lapse of several months between operations, in the event that lacrimal deficiency is a factor. Finally, the patient should be as completely as possible informed of the complications of this surgery.

Following the placement of a protective lens over the globe and the injection of adequate local anesthetic, the lid is everted on a lid clamp and a small area over the superior lateral border of the tarsus is horizontally incised (Plate 11-1, A).

With a blunt scissors, the tissue is dissected to the level of the palpebral portion of the lacrimal gland, a firm, pinkish gray tissue that is prolapsed downward. The gland is grasped with a forceps and excised (Plate 11-1, B). It is sent for pathologic confirmation.

The conjunctiva is then closed with two or three multiple 6-0 chromic catgut sutures (Plate 11-1, C). A light dressing is applied and then removed after 24 hours, Artificial tears are used for several days postoperatively. If dryness occurs, the first attempt should be to close one punctum.

Plate 11-1

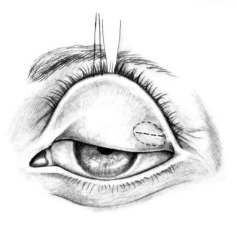

A, A small incision at the upper tarsal border of the everted upper lid.

B, The palpebral portion of the lacrimal gland is excised.

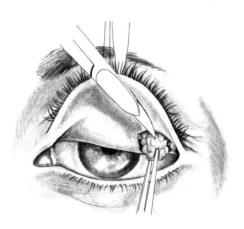

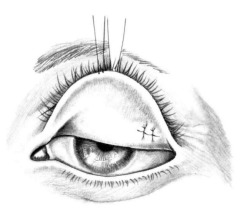

C, Conjunctiva closed with interrupted absorbable sutures.

The palpebral portion of the lacrimal gland often prolapses downward, since it is not firmly supported. It can usually be seen if one everts the upper lid in the elderly patient. The orbital part of the gland, posterior to the orbital septum, is more firmly enclosed. However, in true blepharochalasis it may also be prolapsed. The displacement of this gland produces a bulge under the lid skin that is clearly visible.

To replace this gland within the lacrimal fossa, an incision is made along the supratarsal crease from the middle to the temporal aspect of the lid (Plate 11-2, *A*). Adequate anesthesia and protection for the globe are provided.

The upper aspect of the incision is dissected deep to the orbicularis and upward to the superior orbital rim. The orbital septum inserting into the rim is now visible (Plate 11-2, *B*).

The preseptal orbicularis is incised 2 mm below the superior orbital rim. It is important to maintain this 2 mm rim for proper closure (Plate 11-2, *C*).

Applying gentle pressure on the globe through the lid causes the pinkish gray lacrimal gland to prolapse (Plate 11-2, *D*). Yellowish orbital fat is usually also present and can be excised if it is excessive.

A biopsy of the gland is routinely performed, and the area is sutured with 5-0 chromic catgut suture. A double-armed 4-0 chromic suture is passed through the anterior aspect of the gland (Plate 11-2, *E*).

Plate 11-2

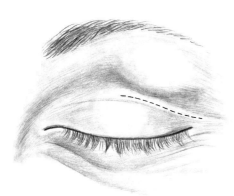

A, Suspension of prolapsed lacrimal gland. Area to be incised is marked at the superior orbital rim.

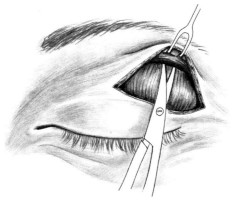

B, The lid is incised, and the dissection is carried down to the orbital septum.

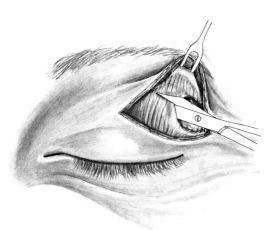

C, The orbital septum is incised.

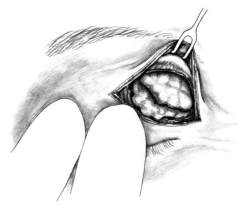

D, The prolapsed lacrimal gland is exposed.

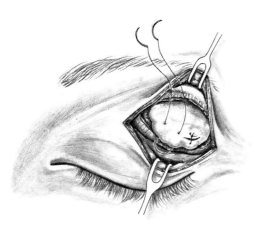

E, A biopsy is performed. A double-armed suture is placed through the gland.

With the gland retracted forward, the two arms of the mattress suture are passed from behind forward in the roof of the lacrimal fossa (Plate 11-2, *F* and *G*).

A nasal speculum can be used to give a view of the fossa. When the suture is tied, it will pull the gland into place within the fossa (Plate 11-2, *H*).

Using interrupted 4-0 chromic catgut sutures, the surgeon closes the septum orbitale (Plate 11-2, *I*). At this point any redundant skin and orbicularis tissue are excised (Plate 11-2, *J*). The wound is closed with interrupted 6-0 silk sutures (Plate 11-2, *K*). A light dressing is applied and then removed after 24 hours. The moderate swelling that results usually subsides after several days. The sutures are removed after 4 days.

Plate 11-2, cont'd

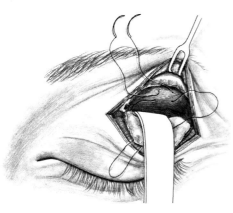

F, The suture is inserted into the roof of the lacrimal fossa.

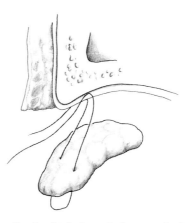

G, Sagittal view of placement of suspension suture.

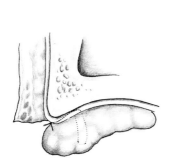

H, Sagittal view of gland suspended in fossa.

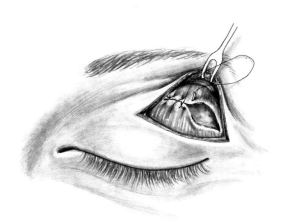

I, Closure of orbital septum.

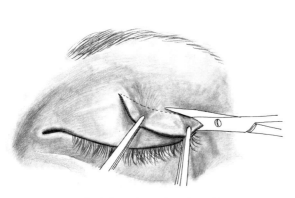

J, Excision of overlapping skin.

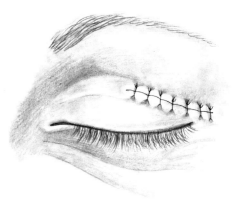

K, Skin closure with interrupted sutures.

CHAPTER 12

DACRYOCYSTORHINOSTOMY OF THE LACRIMAL EXCRETORY SYSTEM

After it has been ascertained, clinically by the presence of mucous or mucopurulent material in the lacrimal sac or following the application of primary and secondary dye tests, that an obstruction exists at the level of the nasolacrimal duct, the procedure of choice is the dacryocystorhinostomy.

A nasal examination is mandatory before consideration of surgery in this area, since the nasolacrimal duct empties below the inferior turbinate. A nasal pathologic condition may possibly be the cause of the obstruction. In addition, radiography of the area should be performed and may reveal a congenital or traumatic obstruction that should be further evaluated. Dacryocystorhinostomy is easy to perform and can yield valuable information, especially regarding the presence of neoplasms in the lacrimal area.

General anesthesia is preferred for this procedure. However, a local anesthetic can be used in adult patients if necessary. The nasal mucosa is injected preoperatively with 1% lidocaine with 1:100,000 epinephrine. The nose is packed with nasal gauze soaked in phenylephrine.

A methylene blue marking pencil is used to designate the area of incision, which begins over the medial canthal tendon and extends along the inferior orbital rim. The length of the incision can be extended as needed (Plate 12-1, *A*). The medial canthus is also injected with a topical anesthetic with epinephrine.

The skin is incised, and a hemostat or a blunt scissors is used to dissect through the orbicularis and subcutaneous tissue down to the periosteum. With retractors in place the periosteum is vertically incised. A periosteal elevator is then used to dissect the lacrimal sac from the lacrimal groove well, and the sac is reflected temporally (Plate 12-1, *B*).

With the anterior lacrimal crest stripped of tissue, a drilling device is used to perforate the anterior lacrimal crest. Irrigation should be maintained while the drill is in use. A suction is helpful during this part of the procedure (Plate 12-1, *C*).

Plate 12-1

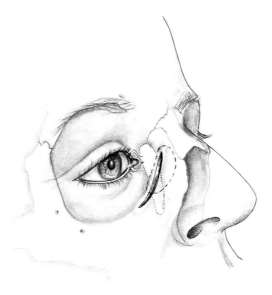

A, Initial incision from medial canthal area along inferior orbital rim, showing relation to lacrimal sac and bony structures.

B, Periosteum is incised and lacrimal sac reflected.

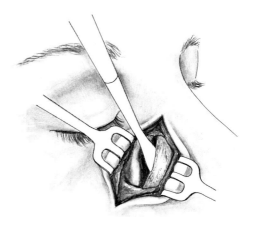

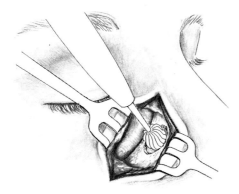

C, Burr used to perforate anterior lacrimal crest.

Front- and side-cutting rongeurs are then used to enlarge the osteotomy. The primary reason for failure of this procedure is the closure of an inadequate osteotomy (Plate 12-1, *D*).

A knife blade is used to incise the nasal mucosa into a vertical **H** shape so that two flaps, one posterior and one anterior, can be prepared. A lacrimal probe is placed through the canaliculus, and the lacrimal sac is identified. The base of the sac is then incised into flaps to oppose those created in the nasal septal mucosa (Plate 12-1, *E*).

The posterior flaps are sutured with two or three interrupted 6-0 chromic catgut sutures. Optimally, a piece of polyethylene tubing is then inserted through the osteotomy and into the nose, where it is sutured into place to maintain the patency of the osteotomy. Alternatively, the nasal packing can be advanced through the osteotomy to serve this purpose (Plate 12-1, *F*).

The anterior flaps are then sutured with 6-0 chromic catgut suture (Plate 12-1, *G*). The retractors are then removed and the subcutaneous tissues closed with 5-0 chromic sutures. The skin is closed with 6-0 silk suture (Plate 12-1, *H*).

A light dressing is applied and then removed after 24 hours. The nasal packing is advanced daily until it can be effortlessly removed, usually after 2 days. The skin sutures are removed after 4 days.

Plate 12-1, cont'd

D, Rongeur used to enlarge osteotomy.

E, Lacrimal sac and nasal cartilage are incised and flaps prepared.

Plate 12-1, cont'd

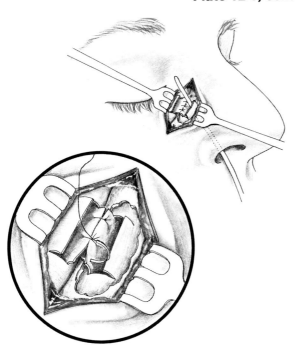

F, Inset shows posterior flaps being sutured. Tubing placed through osteotomy and into nose.

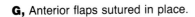

G, Anterior flaps sutured in place.

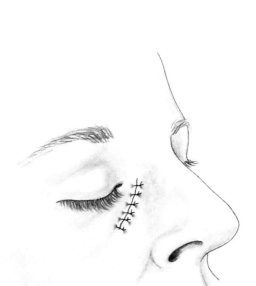

H, Skin closure with interrupted sutures.

CHAPTER 13

BLEPHAROPTOSIS

The preoperative evaluation of the ptosis patient is probably as significant to the treatment of this condition as is the type of surgery and skill with which it is performed. One must begin by differentiating between acquired and congenital ptosis. An accurate history must be taken, and it should be documented by photography if possible. The preoperative photographs should be taken with the eyes in all positions of gaze. The amount of ptosis surgery required for congenital ptosis is greater than that required for acquired ptosis; performing an unsuitable procedure will lead to a less than satisfactory postoperative result.

A complete ophthalmologic examination must be performed, and it must include a careful study of muscle balance to rule out the possibility of a hypotropia causing a pseudoptosis. A Schirmer test for adequacy of lacrimal production should be performed in case an overcorrection results, even transiently.

An estimate should be made of levator function by measuring the interpalpebral fissure in primary position, in upward and downward gaze. During these measurements the action of the frontalis muscle should be inhibited by exerting external pressure on the brow. Patients with good levator function generally require less correction than those patients with less than 5 mm of levator function. In congenital ptosis with less than 3 mm of levator function, a frontalis suspension probably produces the best results.

The patient should be tested for adequate Bell's phenomenon. Good elevation of the globe during forced closure of the lids is a good sign that any postoperative lagophthalmos that occurs will be well tolerated.

The patient should be examined for congenital or traumatic fibrosis in the upper lid. A lagophthalmos on down-gaze with a mechanical obstruction to active extension of the lid will mean further lagophthalmos if ptosis surgery is performed.

A patient may have an apparent ptosis in one eye as compared to the other when the apparently normal eye is actually proptosed. The possibility of this should be kept in mind and properly evaluated.

The presence of a Marcus Gunn phenomenon or a jaw-winking phenomenon should be ascertained by history or observation. Failure to note this relatively common condition in ptosis patients could have disastrous consequences.

The neurologic status of the patient should be checked if necessary. Edrophonium (Tensilon) testing for ocular myasthenia may be indicated. Neurogenic ptosis resulting from third nerve injury usually requires frontalis suspension.

Finally, it should be explained to the patient or parent that ptosis surgery is more an art than a calculable science and that, even in the best of hands, complications can and do result.

Of the many ptosis procedures available in the literature, the three we find most practical in handling almost all cases of ptosis are (1) the frontalis fixation, (2) the external levator resection, and (3) the Fasanella-Servat procedure.

In those cases in which resection or advancement of the levator aponeurosis is not indicated, as in external ophthalmoplegia, congenital ptosis with minimal levator function, aberrant nerve regeneration, or mechanical restriction of the lid, the suspension of the lid margin from the frontalis muscle is a reliable if not the cosmetically preferable method of correction. Even in those cases with poor or absent Bell's phenomenon resulting from extraocular muscle restriction or paresis, this procedure is usually well tolerated, and offers the advantage of simple removal of the supporting sutures if desired. In recent years we have performed a large number of these procedures using 4-0 Supramid suture swaged onto a ski needle, and only rarely have we had to remove the suture in cases of wound infection or granuloma. Fascia lata, now available commercially, is also an excellent material for use in this procedure. The configuration we prefer for this procedure is the double rhomboid, and it is probably that which is used by most surgeons performing this surgery.

With the patient under general anesthesia, three stab incisions are made with a knife blade above the brow in the central, medial, and lateral areas. Then, with adequate protection for the globe, preferably a bone plate, three incisions are made about 2 mm above the lash line and down to the tarsus.

The ski needle with the swaged-on 4-0 Supramid is then inserted through the temporal incision and moved downward to be withdrawn from the lateral lid incision (Plate 13-1, A). The needle is reinserted and moved medially, where it is withdrawn from the central incision. It is then passed superiorly and withdrawn from the central incision above the brow. Finally, it is reinserted into this incision and is withdrawn from the original temporal site. A similar rhomboid is created on the medial aspect of the lid, the central incisions being utilized a second time.

The sutures are then tied in the superior temporal and superior nasal sites, and by adjusting the tension of the suture the surgeon can determine the height of the lid. The knots are inserted into the depth of the wound, and the lid assumes its new position (Plate 13-1, B). The superior superficial incisions are closed with interrupted 6-0 silk sutures. The procedure is repeated on the contralateral upper lid.

A light dressing is applied and then removed after 24 hours. Artificial tears are used every hour postoperatively with a bland ointment instilled at night. The patient generally tolerates the procedure well, and it is rare that the superficial sutures need taking down.

Plate 13-1

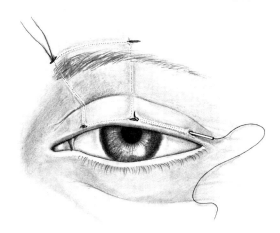

A, Ski needle used to carry Supramid suture through stab incisions.

B, Completion of double rhomboid–type fixation.

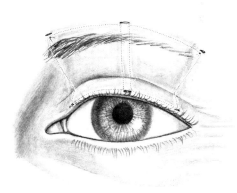

The anterior approach to resection or advancement of the levator aponeurosis has been shown to be an excellent procedure in cases of acquired or congenital ptosis. The exposure of the aponeurosis in congenital ptosis is unsurpassed by any other procedure and permits resection and tarsal advancement enough to correct almost any amount of ptosis. In acquired ptosis, whether from involutional slippage of the aponeurosis, traumatic dehiscence, or myogenic weakness, it allows the lid to be set at any desired level with easy and directly visible accessibility to all of the lid structures.

General anesthesia is used for children of course; for traumatic muscle repair or advancement to an original insertion in adults, the local injection of 2% lidocaine with 1:100,000 epinephrine permits the correction to be gauged in the operating room. Through experience we have found that in cases of acquired senile ptosis it is best to seek a slight overcorrection; otherwise, the lid level will fall after several months.

A contact shell is generally placed over the globe for protection (Plate 13-2, A).

A cotton-tipped applicator is used to elevate the lid margin and estimate the level of the supratarsal crease, which is often absent in cases of ptosis (Plate 13-2, B).

The supratarsal crease is then designated with a marking pencil. The area is infiltrated with a local anesthetic regardless of the type of anesthestic used, because it provides hydraulic dissection of the skin from the orbicularis and aids in hemostasis, as well as producing akinesia (Plate 13-2, C).

With the lid stretched, a razor blade knife is used to incise the designated area, which is dissected inferiorly between the skin and orbicularis to just above the lash line (Plate 13-2, D).

The razor blade knife is then used to undermine a narrow strip of skin along the superior edge of the wound while a forceps holds the lid taut (Plate 13-2, E).

Plate 13-2

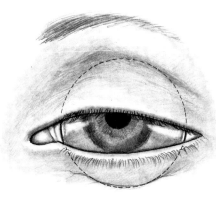

A, Ptotic lid with contact shell before surgery.

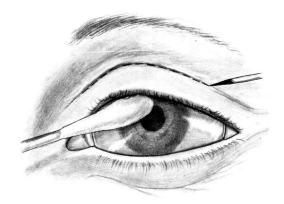

B, Lid margin lifted with cotton applicator and supratarsal crease outlined.

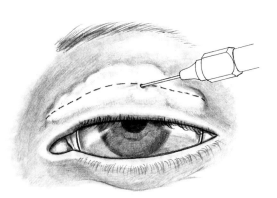

C, Subcutaneous infiltration of anesthetic for lid akinesia and hydraulic dissection.

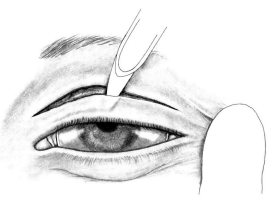

D, Lid is incised and skin undermined to lid margin.

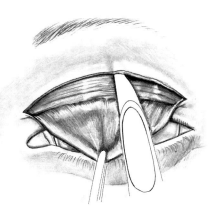

E, Undermining skin down to orbicularis along upper margin of incision.

Skin hooks or a forceps is then used to grasp the lower skin flap, and with the lid on stretch the pretarsal orbicularis is incised at its temporal aspect and undermined to separate it from the underlying tarsus. A transverse incision is made above the lash roots, and the pretarsal orbicularis is excised (Plate 13-2, *F*).

Just above the superior temporal aspect of the exposed tarsus, the tissue is perforated with scissors. A straight hemostat is inserted with one blade on each side of the lid. The lower blade again perforates the lid, this time in its superomedial aspect, and the clamp is closed. The hemostat is now just above the superior border of the tarsus and contains within it conjunctiva, Müller's fibers, and levator aponeurosis (Plate 13-2, *G*).

With the lid now in a normal position, a scissors is used to perforate the orbital septum (Plate 13-2, *H*). If the incision has been made in the correct plane, the white sheath of the aponeurosis is visible with preaponeurotic fat lying above it. Dissection is carried horizontally in both directions. Along the inferior border of the hemostat, a knife blade is used to sever all of the tissue contained in the clamp from the top of the tarsus (Plate 13-2, *I*). Vertical incisions are then created at the ends of this incision and extended up into the fornices. These incisions must not be angled but made straight back.

Plate 13-2, cont'd

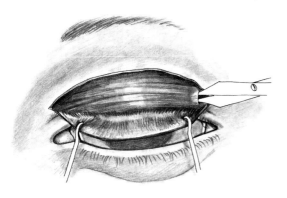

F, Pretarsal orbicularis undermined and excised to expose tarsal plate.

G, Lid is everted and clamp inserted along border of tarsus.

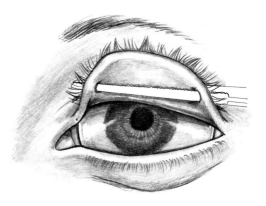

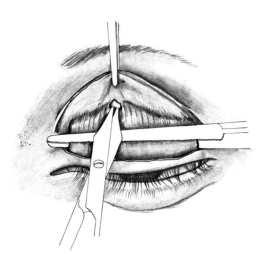

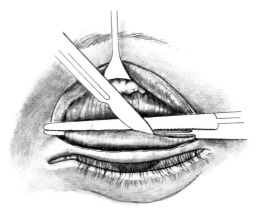

I, Preaponeurotic fat is exposed and levator aponeurosis apparent. Full-thickness incision is made along upper tarsal border.

H, Orbital septum incised.

With the clamp elevated, the conjunctiva is ballooned away from Müller's fibers. It is carefully dissected free from the muscle layer (Plate 13-2, *J*).

With a continuous 6-0 absorbable suture the conjunctiva is replaced at the top of the tarsus (Plate 13-2, *K*).

A double-armed 5-0 chromic suture is then placed in the midtarsus to a depth of about one half the tarsal plate. The double-armed suture is then brought through the clamped tissues, at a level just above the area to be resected. The contact shell and the clamp are then removed (Plate 13-2, *L* and *M*).

Plate 13-2, cont'd

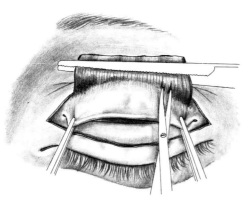

J, Conjunctiva dissected free from Müller's muscle.

K, Conjunctiva closed with absorbable suture.

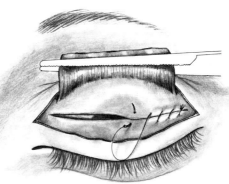

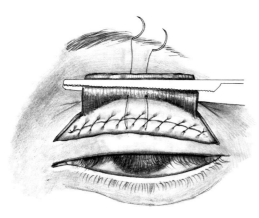

L, Double-armed midtarsal suture placed and passed through levator aponeurosis.

M, Sagittal section of lid to demonstrate placement of midtarsal suture.

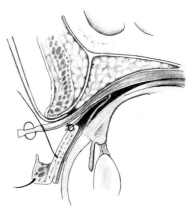

The suture is tightened but not tied, and the lid level is evaluated. This lid margin should be just below the superior limbus. If the lid is not at the desired level, the suture is removed and reinserted until the proper level is reached (Plate 13-2, *N*). The suture is tied, and two more double-armed 5-0 chromic catgut sutures are placed, one medially and one laterally. The excess levator is measured and excised (Plate 13-2, *O*).

For skin closure three 6-0 chromic sutures are placed full thickness through the superior skin edge to grasp the levator aponeurosis and exit through the inferior skin edge. This creates an excellent lid fold and does not require suture removal in children (Plate 13-2, *P*).

Postoperatively, especially in congenital ptosis, patients should be observed for corneal irritation caused by lagophthalmos and treated accordingly with artificial tears and bland ointments.

In the event of undercorrection, the procedure should be repeated. If the levator function was poor to begin with, a frontalis fixation eventually may be necessary.

If an overcorrection has resulted, massage of the lid and exercise of the orbicular function are useful. If this combined with eventual adaptation of the eye to the new lid level fails, the best solution is to perform a recession of the levator to a higher point in the tarsus or even with the substitution of banked sclera between the levator and the tarsus.

Plate 13-2, cont'd

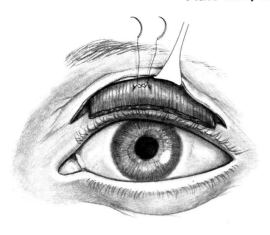

N, Suture tied and lid level evaluated.

O, Dissection of excess levator.

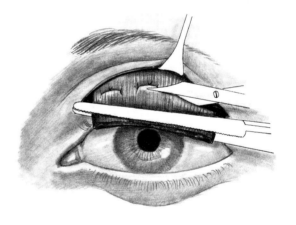

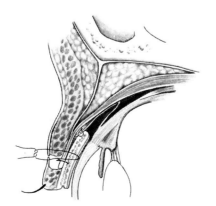

P, Sagittal section to illustrate lid closure.

In cases of minimal ptosis in which the function of the levator is good and the ptosis does not exceed 2 mm, the Fasanella-Servat procedure is useful.

With adequate protection for the globe and local anesthesia obtained with 2% lidocaine with 1:100,000 epinephrine, the upper lid is everted and two curved hemostats are placed, one medially and one temporally. A 6-0 double-armed monofilament suture is passed full thickness from the external surface of the lid to just under the temporal hemostat (Plate 13-3, A and B).

Within the hemostats are contained the conjunctiva, the upper lid retractors, and the superior edge of the tarsus.

The suture is threaded back and forth behind the clamps at a 45-degree angle, with the exit site used as the entrance for the next needle pass (Plate 13-3, C and D). At the medial end of the everted lid, the suture exits through full thickness to the external surface of the lid (Plate 13-3, E).

Plate 13-3

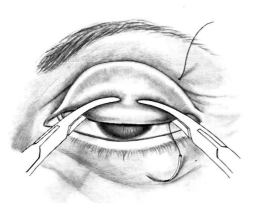

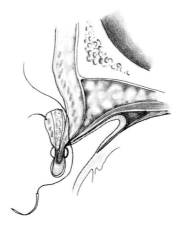

A, Lid everted and curved hemostats placed.

B, Sagittal view of initial suture placement before weaving technique.

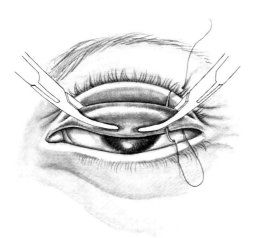

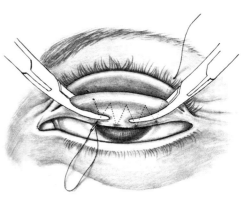

C. Monofilament suture passed full thickness through supratarsal crease to below clamp.

D, Suture woven in back of clamp.

E, Suture through full thickness of lid.

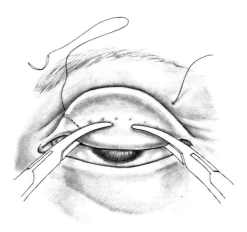

The tissue in front of the clamp is excised (Plate 13-3, *F*).

The monofilament suture is tied on top of the lid. A light dressing is applied. The suture is removed after 1 week (Plate 13-3, *G*).

We have thus far had no problems with this technique. Since the needle enters and exits from the same site, there is no suture exposed to the cornea on the underside of the lid.

Plate 13-3, cont'd

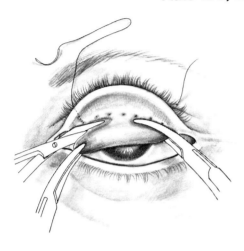

F, Resection of tissue in front of clamp.

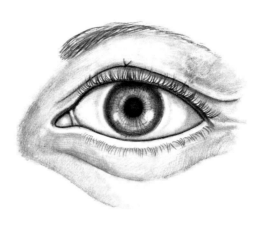

G, Suture tied in place.

CHAPTER 14

SYMBLEPHARON

Progressive inflammatory disease such as pemphigoid and erythema multiforme, old traumatic injuries, and chemical injuries such as alkali burns all tend to produce continual scarring and contracture of the conjunctiva, with destruction of all of its lubricating elements and a resultant entropion of both upper and lower lids. There is a gradual obliteration of the cul-de-sacs, and the resulting dryness causes corneal damage with opacity and vascularization of the cornea. Procedures such as Z-plasty, conjunctival transplantation, and the placement of scleral rings, while they may provide temporary relief, are eventually overcome by the unrelenting disease process. A procedure that we have used for these severe and desperate cases involves large mucous membrane grafts to re-form the cul-de-sacs and a lid-splitting technique as a cure for the entropion.

Because of the extensive dissection involved and the need for large buccal mucous membrane grafts to be taken, re-formation of cul-de-sacs is best performed with the patient under general anesthesia.

Sutures of 6-0 silk are passed through the center of the medial and temporal third of the upper and lower lid margins. The lids are then maximally retracted.

A Bard-Parker blade is used to dissect the scarred conjunctiva and free the lids from the adherent sclera (Plate 14-1, A). Profuse bleeding usually occurs. Continuous irrigation is most helpful during this dissection, whereas the injection of local anesthetic with epinephrine is to no avail. Moderate pressure and vasoconstrictors are applied when the dissection is complete. Cautery should be avoided since this is a graft bed.

Lysis of the conjunctival bands is continued until the area of the recti insertions is reached. Care is taken not to damage these.

Split-thickness mucous membrane grafts are taken from the mouth, to be used as a lining for the cul-de-sacs. A Castroviejo mucotome set at 0.5 mm is used to obtain the donor grafts. The area from which the graft is to be taken is injected with 1% lidocaine with 1:100,000 epinephrine. In these cases it is usually necessary to utilize both upper and lower lids, as well as the mucosa of the cheeks. As each graft is taken, it is transferred to the recipient site, where it is meticulously sutured with 7-0 chromic catgut suture, the raw surface toward the globe (Plate 14-1, B).

The perilimbal area is sutured first. Because split-thickness grafts contract considerably, they should not be sutured in a stretched position. Finally, full-thickness 6-0 silk mattress sutures are placed in the fornices and tied over cotton bolsters on the external surface of the lids (Plate 14-1, C).

A scleral shell with the central area removed is placed over the globe, and the lids are sutured closed. The marginal sutures are removed after several days; however, the scleral shell is left in position until the graft has healed in place.

Following an interval of 4 to 6 weeks, it is possible to attempt to repair the entropion.

Plate 14-1

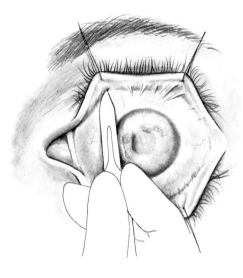

A, Adherent lids dissected from sclera.

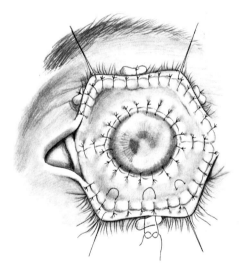

B, Mucous membrane grafts sutured into position.

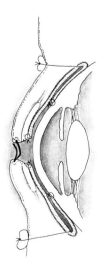

C, Sagittal section to illustrate placement of sutures in cul-de-sacs.

A razor blade knife is used to make an incision at the mucocutaneous junction of the upper and lower lids, splitting the lids into two lamellae. The incision is carried laterally from an area temporal to the punctum almost to the lateral canthus (Plate 14-2, *A*).

The dissection is continued deep enough into each lid that 5 mm of posterior lamella can be advanced. The advanced lamellae are sutured together with continuous 5-0 chromic catgut. The lid margins are recessed and sutured to the upper portion of the advanced lamellae with interrupted 6-0 chromic sutures (Plate 14-2, *B* and *C*).

Plate 14-2

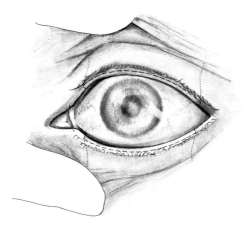

A, Horizontal midmarginal tarsal incision and external incisions outlined.

B, Internal lamellae advanced and sutured into place.

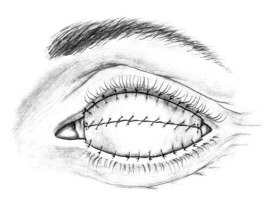

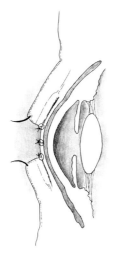

C, Sagittal view to illustrate advancement and suturing of internal lamallae. Note recession of lid margins.

A full-thickness (1 mm) mucous membrane graft is obtained freehand from the area of the lower lip to fit over the area created by the posterior lamellae. This is sutured into place with interrupted 6-0 chromic catgut sutures (Plate 14-2, *D*).

After a period of 2 months, to allow for healing and detumescence of the tissue, the graft is opened. The lid margins regress and hypertrophy over several months (Plate 14-2, *E*).

Plate 14-2, cont'd

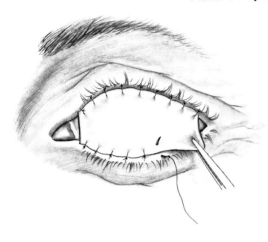

D, Full-thickness mucous membrane graft sutured into place.

E, Tarsorrhaphy opened after 8 weeks.

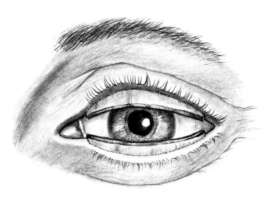

CHAPTER 15

RECURRENT PTERYGIA

The treatment for recurrent or hypertrophic pterygia, once it has been ascertained that one is dealing with a benign condition, is the adequate resection of the involved tissue and the placement of normal tissue in the area to act as an anatomic barrier.

Following the injection of a local anesthetic into the lids by the modified Van Lint method, a lid speculum is placed into position to provide adequate exposure of the globe.

The pterygium is gently grasped with a fixation forceps, and a solution of 1% lidocaine with 1:100,000 epinephrine is injected into the tissue superficial to the corneal stroma. This not only provides akinesia but also facilitates dissection (Plate 15-1, *A*).

With a razor blade knife, dissection is initiated at the apex of the lesion. A superficial keratectomy is performed, and the pterygium is dissected back over the limbus onto the episclera (Plate 15-1, *B*). With the pterygium stretched, the dissection is carried to the insertion of the medial rectus muscle. All involved tissue is then resected, with care taken not to injure the muscle insertion.

A solution of 1% lidocaine with 1:100,000 epinephrine is injected subconjunctivally under the tissue of the temporal aspect of the globe.

Plate 15-1

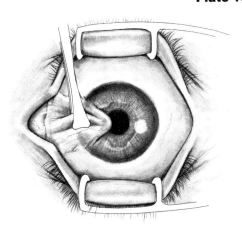

A, Pterygium occupying nasal aspect of cornea.

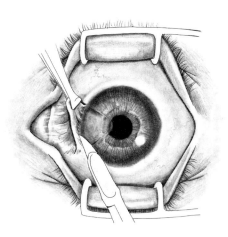

B, Dissection of pterygium from cornea and sclera.

A crescentic incision is made about 1 mm from the limbus from the 12 o'clock to the 6 o'clock position. A second concentric incision is created 5 mm temporal to this (Plate 15-1, *C*).

The flap is left attached at each extremity, but it is dissected free in the central portion.

The recipient bed should now be carefully dissected free of any fibrotic material and then excised. Hemostasis is achieved by applying pressure and by vasoconstrictors, as in any graft bed.

The conjunctival flap is then carefully transposed to the new site. Sutures of 7-0 chromic catgut are placed to orient the flap in several areas. This accomplished, meticulous suturing should continue until the flap is evenly secured in place. The bases of the flap are not sutured, because any redundant tissue here will flatten over a several-week period (Plate 15-1, *D*).

The donor site is likewise closed with interrupted sutures of 7-0 chromic catgut. The site will generally close with minimal tension. However, a scleral hook is useful in bringing together the ends of the tissue during suturing (Plate 15-1, *E*).

A light dressing is applied and is changed daily for several days. No ophthalmic ointment is used.

In the postoperative period the transplanted area vascularizes along the arc of the graft; this inhibits horizontal regrowth of the pterygium.

Plate 15-1, cont'd

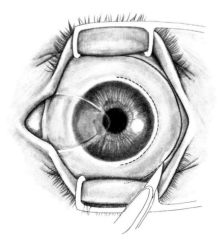

C, Conjunctival flap prepared.

D, Conjunctival flap transposed and
   sutured into place.

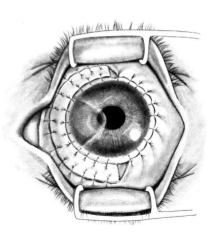

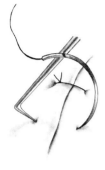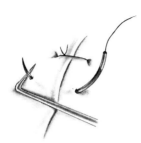

E, Scleral hook used during suture
   insertion.

CHAPTER 16

SOCKET RECONSTRUCTION

In those cases in which contracture of tissues in the anophthalmic socket has made even the most skillful fitting of a prosthetic device an impossibility, the surgeon must replace the deficiency of tissue with a suitable substitute. Commonly seen in cases involving inflammatory disease, traumatic injury, tissue avulsion, chemical burns, and faulty enucleation technique and following involutional fibrotic change, a contracted socket results from a shortening or shrinkage of the tissue in the orbit.

The surgeon has several choices for repairing the defect. Mucous membrane grafts can be used in cases in which the contracture is mild and limited. The techniques of taking these grafts and inserting them will be described. For more extensive cases a split-thickness skin graft can be used to line the entire socket.

In some cases the original implant will have extruded or migrated. In these cases we have successfully used a composite dermis-fat graft not only to replace the implant but also to increase the dimension of the socket.

General anesthesia is preferred for mucous membrane grafts.

Following the placement of 6-0 silk sutures at the centers of the medial and temporal thirds of the upper and lower lids to act as traction sutures, a Bard-Parker blade is used to horizontally incise the contracted conjunctival tissue (Plate 16-1, A). The injection of a local anesthetic with epinephrine is of limited value in achieving hemostasis but in some cases does aid in hydraulic dissection.

A sharp scissors is used to undermine the conjunctival tissue. It is useful to grasp the tissue edges with skin hooks and exert traction in the opposite direction of the dissection. The conjunctiva is dissected inferiorly first and then superiorly to the lid margin. Special care is taken in the upper lid dissection to not injure the upper lid retractors (Plate 16-1, B).

A horizontal incision is then made over the inferior orbital rim. The incision should be made full thickness down to the bone. The rim is palpated and can be used as a guide and support. A hemostat is used to spread the surrounding tissue and allow good exposure of the bony rim. A drilling device is then used to create a full-thickness hole in the inferior orbital rim (Plate 16-1, B).

With skin hooks used to retract the conjunctival lining, the subconjunctival fibrotic tissue in the socket should be excised to allow placement of a conformer. Once again, any dissection in the superior cul-de-sac should be done with care to not disrupt the levator muscle or its aponeurosis. The inferior dissection should be as close as possible to the hole drilled through the inferior orbital rim (Plate 16-1, C).

Plate 16-1

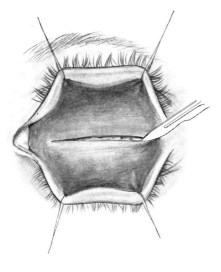

A, Lids retracted and horizontal incision made.

B, Lining of socket dissected and hole drilled through inferior orbital rim.

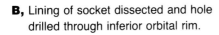

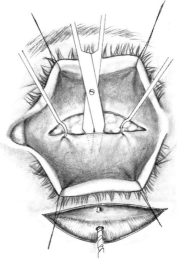

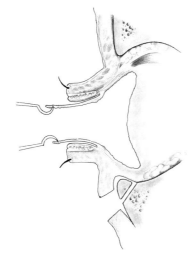

C, Sagittal view of new socket.

A conformer is then molded to the socket. The material we prefer is dental molding compound, which can be softened in warm water and molded with no great difficulty in the operating room. The edges of the conformer should be smooth and the center drilled out so that an 8 to 10 mm opening is present to facilitate fluid drainage.

In the inferior portion of the doughnut-shaped conformer, another smaller hole should be drilled, which will come into proximity to the hole drilled in the inferior orbital rim.

The mucous membrane graft should be relatively thick (0.8 mm). The lower lip is everted and held in position with an appropriate clamp or towel hooks. The mucosa is injected with 1% lidocaine with 1:100,000 epinephrine. In these areas the surgeon uses a razor blade knife instead of a mucotome to take a freehand graft, so that he is certain to obtain a reasonably thick graft. Split-thickness grafts will contract up to 50%. The donor site need not be sutured, but will freely granulate.

The mucous membrane is folded over the conformer with the raw surface outward (Plate 16-1, *D*). It is then placed in the dissected cavity so that the raw surface is in contact with the newly dissected area. The mucous membrane graft is sutured with moderate tension to the conformer lining with absorbable suture. The conformer is then removed and perforated at the center for drainage.

If the area to be re-formed is large, split-thickness skin from a smooth area of the body is obtained with a mechanical dermatome. It is used in a similar fashion.

A fine stainless steel wire is then threaded through the hole in the inferior orbital rim and passed through the socket and out between the lids. The wire is passed through the graft and the smaller inferior hole in the conformer. The conformer is threaded into place in the socket. The wire is then secured in place by twisting it with a hemostat and it is brought into apposition with the inferior orbital rim. The end is clipped with a wire cutter and rotated to remain within the conformer.

The incision overlying the inferior orbital rim is closed in layered fashion, with 5-0 chromic catgut used to close the subcutaneous layer and interrupted sutures of 6-0 silk used to close the skin (Plate 16-1, *E*).

Interpalpebral sutures of 6-0 silk are placed, which together with the stainless steel wire will hold the conformer in place (Plate 16-1, *F*).

The skin and interpalpebral sutures are removed after 4 days. A light dressing is changed daily for several days. Postoperatively, topical antibiotics are used.

The conformer is left in place for approximately 4 to 6 weeks, at which time the wire is cut and the conformer removed. A temporary conformer is placed in position until a prosthetic device can be fitted.

Plate 16-1, cont'd

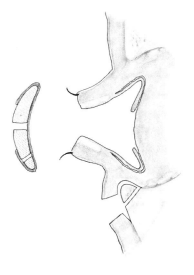

D, Conformer shaped to fit new socket and conformer lined with mucous membrane.

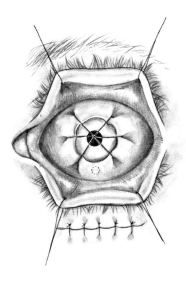

E, Conformer sutured into place and skin incision closed.

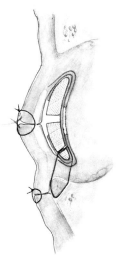

F, Sagittal view to illustrate conformer wired into position.

DERMIS-FAT GRAFTS

(Plate 16-2)

The use of autogenous dermis-fat grafts as a replacement for migrated or extruding orbital implants has proven to be an excellent method for secondary replacement of these primary synthetic implants.

A variety of materials have been used for orbital implants: sclera, fascia lata, and temporal fascia. The extrusion or migration of orbital implants is a common complication of enucleation. Not only does it produce a cosmetic defect but also the recurrent exposure and infection of tissue cause a contraction of the socket. The added benefit of dermis-fat grafting is an increase in the dimension of the socket.

When the patient has a migrated and/or partially extruding orbital implant, one is generally able to palpate the implant through the closed lid to ascertain its location (Plate 16-2, A). This should be done preoperatively and noted. Later, with the patient in the supine position in the operating room, this is more difficult.

General anesthesia is required for this procedure. A lid speculum (or 6-0 silk traction sutures) is placed in the eye to give adequate exposure. If the implant is extruding, the area of conjunctival erosion is visible (Plate 16-2, B). We generally enter from this area and extend the incision from here.

Dissection is carried down through Tenon's capsule into the area in which the implant lies. The implant is isolated and removed. If the implant is not within the central cavity, an attempt is made to locate it (Plate 16-2, C).

After removal of the implant, an attempt is made to locate the muscle stumps that have retracted into the orbit. A forceps is inserted into the sheath in which the muscles lie, and after the stumps have been located they are grasped with hemostats (Plate 16-2, D).

Sutures of 4-0 chromic catgut are then passed through the rectus muscles at the 12, 3, 6, and 9 o'clock positions (Plate 16-2, E).

Plate 16-2

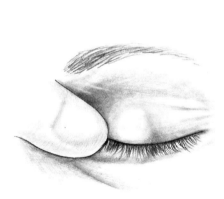

A, Position of extruding or migrating implant palpated through lid.

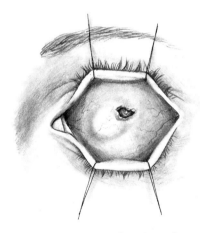

B, Implant extruding through conjunctiva.

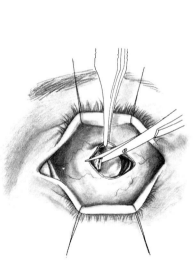

C, Dissection extended down to isolate implant.

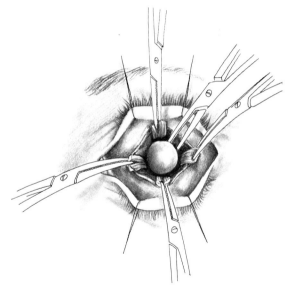

D, Area of horizontal rectus muscles grasped and implant removed.

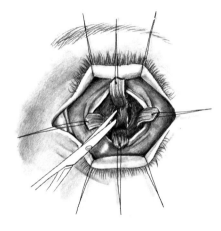

E, Sutures passed through muscle stumps.

Next, attention is turned to the lateral aspect of the thigh near the buttocks, which is prepared and marked for incision (Plate 16-2, *F*). A handheld derma-brader is used to abrade and deepithelialize an area of about 8 by 10 cm. The end point is reached when active bleeding occurs (Plate 16-2, *G*).

The graft is fashioned with a Bard-Parker blade to fit the size of the defect to be filled. Generally, a circumference of about 1.5 cm is sufficient. Because this area of the body has an abundant amount of subcutaneous fat, it is not difficult to remove about 4 cm of fat with the dermis (Plate 16-2, *H*).

Plate 16-2, cont'd

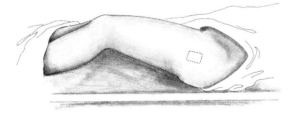

F, Area from which dermis-fat graft is to be taken.

G, Area deepithelialized with handheld dermabrader.

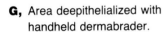

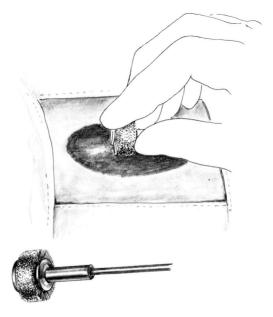

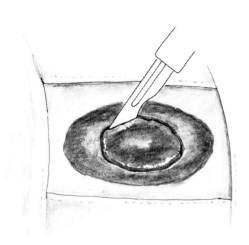

H, Dermis-fat graft excised.

We generally close the donor site in a layered fashion with buried sutures of 4-0 chromic catgut and interrupted superficial sutures of 5-0 silk (Plate 16-2, *I*). The silk sutures are removed after 1 week, and the area reepithelializes in about a month. It is also possible to use near-far, far-near sutures to close the defect, because this two-layered closure will eliminate dead space.

The dermis-fat graft is gently transferred to the recipient bed. No irrigation is used in inserting the graft (Plate 16-2, *J*).

The 4-0 chromic sutures holding the rectus muscles are then sutured directly to the dermis. These four critical sutures hold the graft in place (Plate 16-2, *K*). Some fat may prolapse from the graft edges, but this can be excised later.

Plate 16-2, cont'd

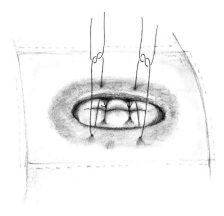

I, Donor site closed.

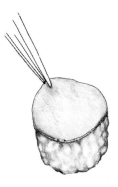

J, Dermis-fat graft to be transferred to socket.

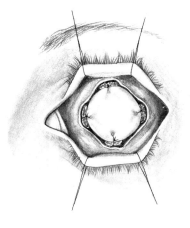

K, Graft first sutured to horizontal rectus muscles.

Additional 4-0 chromic sutures are then placed in interrupted fashion in each quadrant while the rectus sutures at the extremity of the quadrant are stretched (Plate 16-2, *L*).

The four quadrants are then successively closed (Plate 16-2, *M*). Closing the wound without use of the traction method is unnecessarily cumbersome.

The dermis is sutured directly to the conjunctiva and Tenon's capsule so that the graft at the completion of the suturing resembles a corneal button sewn into place (Plate 16-2, *N*).

A doughnut-shaped conformer is then placed in the socket, where it remains until a prosthetic eye is fitted in 2 to 3 weeks. The conjunctival epithelium grows over the graft in 1 month (Plate 16-2, *O*).

A light dressing is applied and changed daily for several days. Postoperatively, antibiotic drops are instilled for several weeks.

The motility obtained with this method is excellent, and recently we have used it as a primary procedure in a limited number of cases.

Plate 16-2, cont'd

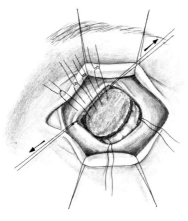
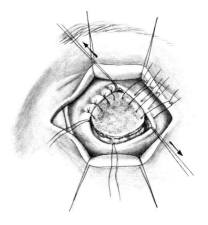

L and **M,** Interrupted sutures used to complete closure as illustrated.

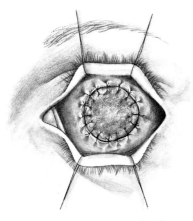
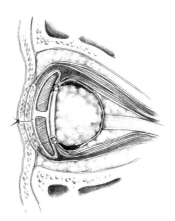

N, Donor graft sutures in place.

O, Sagittal view with conformer in place.

CHAPTER 17

ORBITAL FRACTURES AND MEDIAL CANTHAL RECONSTRUCTION

Orbital fractures can generally be divided into two broad categories: blow-out fractures of the orbital floor (or walls) and fractures involving the orbital rim. Included in the latter category are naso-orbital fractures.

An external force striking the orbital rim meets the strong bony abutment of the orbital region, which generally protects the orbit and its contents from damage other than swelling and ecchymosis of the soft tissue (Plate 17-1, *A*). However, if the impact of the force is on the lids and globe, the orbital contents are retro-pulsed, with a sudden increase in intraorbital pressure, and as a result the thin portion of the orbital floor and/or medial wall is fractured (Plate 17-1, *B*). This is a blow-out fracture of the orbit. These fractures are usually caused by blunt objects greater in diameter than the orbital rim. Fracture of the orbital rim may also occur, in which case one must treat both entities.

Some cases may be very complicated in which the orbital floor has been frac-tured and the contents of the orbit, bone fragments, and tissue adjacent to the inferior oblique and inferior rectus muscles have prolapsed into the maxillary sinus. In other cases the damage is not as extensive and symptoms are caused by swelling around these tissues, which may restrict movement of the muscles. In medial wall fractures there is the possibility of entrapment of the medial rectus muscle.

Functionally, the vertical muscle imbalance secondary to the swelling or entrapment of the tissues near the inferior rectus or inferior oblique muscle is the greatest problem, along with enophthalmos caused by the prolapse of tissue from the orbital cavity or enlargement of the cavity itself. The diplopia that occurs secondary to the vertical muscle imbalance ceases with the restoration of proper ocular movement. One must keep in mind the possibility of direct injury to the motor nerve supply or to the muscles themselves as a cause for delayed resolution of symptoms.

Generally, blow-out fractures cause little damage to the globe itself. If visual loss occurs and slit lamp and funduscopic examinations have shown negative results, one must check for hemorrhage, edema, or fracture at the orbital apex or occlusion of the vascular supply to the optic nerve or retina. On evaluation gen-erally it is noted that the globe is sunken with a deep superior sulcus. The area supplied by the infraorbital nerve often has lost sensation. A forced duction test should be performed, although a positive result may only signify the presence of edema, hemorrhage, or fat entrapment.

The transcutaneous approach is the one we prefer for surgical correction. With the patient under general anesthesia, a methylene blue marking pencil is used to indicate a subciliary incision 3 mm below the lash line from just under the punctum to the lateral smile crease.

The globe is protected with a contact shell. A 6-0 silk suture is passed through the lid margin of the lower lid, and the lid is pulled upward. Often 1% lidocaine with 1:100,000 epinephrine is injected subcutaneously to aid in this dissection.

A razor blade knife is then used to incise the designated area. The skin and orbicularis are undermined with blunt scissors. The incision is extended down along the orbital septum (with care not to perforate this structure) to the perios-teum of the inferior orbital rim. A retractor is used to expose the area. A Bard-Parker blade is used to incise the periosteum about 2 mm below the edge of the inferior orbital rim. Then a periosteal elevator is used to dissect between perios-

Plate 17-1

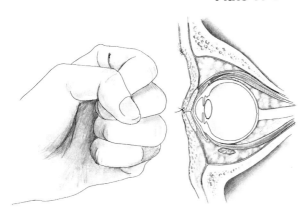

A, External force about to strike orbital area.

B, Increase in intraorbital pressure causes fracture of orbital floor.

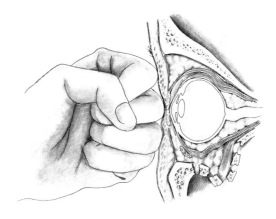

teum and bone upward over the edge of the rim, with the undermining continued into the orbit. When the orbital contents that have herniated through the fracture site are encountered, it is often difficult to free them. The end-on-end use of two blunted periosteal elevators is often helpful. If the orbital contents are still entrapped, it is sometimes necessary to use a hemostat to fracture the edge of the defect to free the entrapped tissue.

The surgeon must be aware of any defects occurring along the medial aspect of the orbital floor. Dissection and inspection of the orbit must include not only the temporal and central aspects of the orbital floor but also this area.

With the orbital contents free, a ribbon retractor is used to elevate the tissue and the implant is placed (Plate 17-1, C).

A variety of synthetic implants can be used to cover the defect in the orbital floor. We generally prefer as thin a piece of material as possible that will hold the contents of the orbit in place. An implant that is too thick will cause further motility problems, and too thin an implant may prolapse into the fracture site.

Although most implants will remain stationary after they have been placed, with the orbital contents resting on them, we often suture the implant to periosteum or create a flap in the anterior surface to prevent forward migration (Plate 17-1, D). The surgeon should also be aware of the posterior extent of the implant. An implant that is placed too deeply in the orbit may compromise circulation or restrict motility.

After the implant is placed and the orbital contents are in proper position, the forced duction test should be repeated to check for adequate support by the implant.

Generally, several interrupted 5-0 chromic sutures are placed to close the periosteum, although these are not absolutely necessary. The muscle and subcutaneous layers are not sutured, because this may cause vertical shortening of the lower lid.

The skin is closed with interrupted sutures of 6-0 silk (Plate 17-1, E). A light dressing is applied.

Cold compresses are applied postoperatively to reduce swelling. Vision is checked 12 hours after the surgery. Dressings are changed daily for several days. The skin sutures are removed after 4 to 5 days.

The postoperative edema that results may cause restriction of motility. This subsides in time, as does the diplopia. If diplopia continues after 6 months, extraocular muscle surgery should be contemplated.

Plate 17-1, cont'd

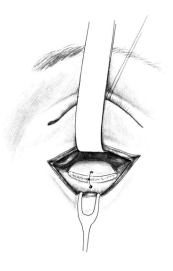

C, Transcutaneous approach with placement of bone in orbital floor.

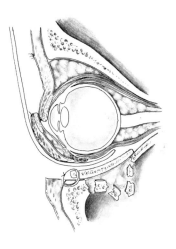

D, Sagittal view of bone implant in place.

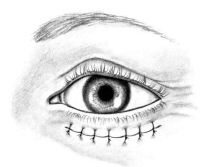

E, Closure of subciliary type of approach.

As a result of a force delivered to the bridge of the nose, the nasal bones are shattered, as well as the frontal process of the maxilla. As the impact continues, the lacrimal and ethmoid bones are fractured and are displaced laterally. The distance between the medial canthi is increased, a condition known as traumatic telecanthus (Plate 17-2, A). Patients with these types of fractures are easy to identify, because they have flattened nasal bridges and displaced medial canthi. If these patients are not seen soon after injury, which is often the case, the bone fragments are then malunited. Along with the destruction of the bony structures, the enclosed components of the lacrimal system are also disrupted.

To repair this area, an open reduction of the fracture with the reconstitution of the lacrimal system via dacryocystorhinostomy is necessary. The canthal tendons are replaced with transnasal wires.

General anesthesia is preferred for this procedure, but nonetheless the area is infiltrated with topical anesthesia containing epinephrine. Nasal packing with gauze soaked in phenylephrine is also preferred at the start of the procedure.

Repair is begun by making a vertical incision about 3 to 5 mm nasal to the medial canthus and dissecting down to the level of the periosteum of the fractured area. The incision is extended as necessary to expose the length of the involved area.

The lacrimal sac is then located. The bone in the area is stripped of periosteum with a periosteal elevator, if possible, and the lacrimal sac is reflected medially. The sac is usually swollen with muco-purulent material.

A mechanical drill is then used to create an osteotomy and at the same time to contour somewhat the medial canthal area (Plate 17-2, B). The lacrimal sac should be given adequate protection during the drilling procedure.

When the nasal mucosa has been reached, flaps are prepared in it and in the lacrimal sac, as has been described for a dacryocystorhinostomy. The posterior flaps are sutured with 5-0 chromic catgut suture (Plate 17-2, C).

Plate 17-2

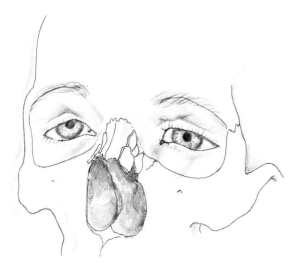

A, Bone displacement in naso-orbital fracture.

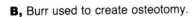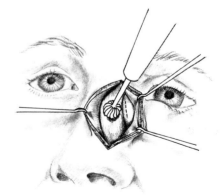

B, Burr used to create osteotomy.

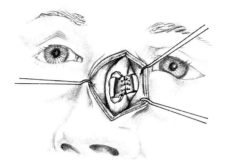

C, Posterior flaps created and sutured between lacrimal sac and lining of nasal bone.

At this point, the procedure is generally repeated on the contralateral side, which is usually involved in these fractures.

The anterior flaps are then sutured with absorbable suture. Next, an air drill is used to drill two holes through the bridge of the nose, one in line with the anterior lacrimal crest and one somewhat posterior, to realign the facial contour (Plate 17-2, *D*).

Stainless steel wires are then passed through the two holes and inserted through the medial canthal tendons on each side. The wires are tightened down to the nasal bridge by twisting them with a hemostat. They are cut with an appropriate wire cutter. The medial canthal tendons have now been repositioned (Plate 17-2, *E*).

Two additional wires are now passed through the holes to emerge through the edges of the skin incision one anterior and one posterior.

Subcutaneous layers are closed with 5-0 chromic catgut suture and the skin with interrupted 6-0 silk sutures. The wire is then threaded through plastic plates and twisted to hold the plates in position against the medial canthus. These plates hold the underlying structures in position and relieve wound tension (Plate 17-2, *F*).

Light dressings are applied and then removed after 24 hours. Cold compresses are applied. The plastic plates are removed after a 2-week period.

Occasionally, nasal reconstruction is required with bone grafts from the iliac crest or ribs. We generally leave this work to a facial plastic or ear, nose, and throat surgeon.

Plate 17-2, cont'd

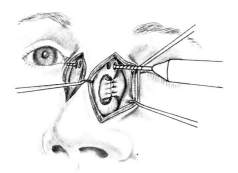

D, Anterior flaps sutured and holes drilled through bridge of nose.

E, Medial canthal tendons wired into position.

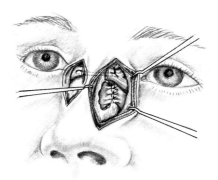

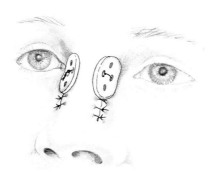

F, Plastic buttons wired into position and incisions closed.

CHAPTER 18

ORBITAL TUMORS

Newer diagnostic techniques have greatly refined the preoperative evaluation of orbital masses. The use of orbital ultrasound and CT scans have made exploration and biopsy necessary in far fewer instances than before. However, it is still often necessary to seek tissue diagnoses to plan further treatment modalities. The diagnosis of a benign lesion may make partial excision or nonsurgical treatment a possibility, whereas a biopsy that suggests a growing mass indicates that more radical treatment is necessary.

Although masses that can be palpated through the lid are usually approachable through a transcutaneous incision, these tumors often extend deeply into the orbit. When these lesions are adherent to the globe or rectus muscles or both, the usual anterior orbital approaches (subciliary, superotemporal, superonasal, and lacrimal) may not offer adequate exposure and accessibility to the tumor. The approach that we prefer for handling tumors of this type is the transmarginal approach, in which the full thickness of the lid is incised to the fornix, affording complete accessibility to the mass (Plate 18-1, *A*). A palpable mass occupying the nasal one third of the upper lid may extend behind the medial canthal tendon (Plate 18-1, *B*) along the globe and medial rectus muscle (Plate 18-1, *C*).

In this procedure we normally prefer general anesthesia, although adequate local anesthesia can be achieved by using 2% lidocaine with 1:100,000 epinephrine.

Plate 18-1

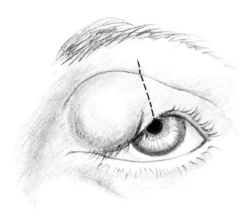

A, Anterior orbital tumor with area of transmarginal incision outlined.

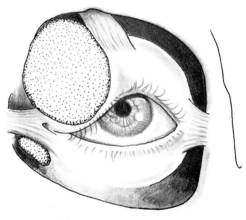

B, Intraorbital extent of tumor.

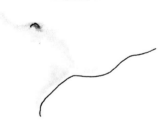

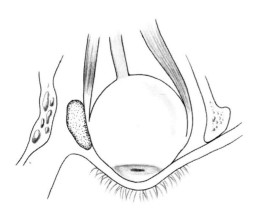

C, Relationship of tumor to medial rectus muscle.

With adequate protection for the globe (usually a lid plate), a full-thickness, vertical transmarginal incision is made with a blunt scissors down to the fornix in the area overlying the mass. To facilitate this incision, both sides of the area outlined for incision are grasped with forceps, and traction is exerted in a downward and outward direction. When the incision has reached the upper fornix, the lid flaps are turned outward and retracted with 4-0 silk sutures passed through the lid margins (Plate 18-1, *D*).

The anterior extent of the tumor is then visible. An incision is made through the conjunctiva from the superior apex of the lid incision, over the tumor mass and into the lower cul-de-sac. Care must be taken to not transversely incise and damage the levator aponeurosis or Müller's muscle in dissecting the tumor.

The mass is grasped with forceps and, while being gently retracted, is bluntly dissected from the underlying sclera and medial rectus muscle (Plate 18-1, *E*).

After the mass has been carefully excised and adequate hemostasis achieved, the conjunctival layer is closed with continuous 6-0 absorbable sutures (Plate 18-1, *F*).

The full-thickness lid incision is closed with the three-suture technique at the lid margin, and the deeper layers are anastomosed with 6-0 absorbable sutures. Interrupted 6-0 silk sutures close the superficial layer (Plate 18-1, *G*).

A light Telfa dressing is applied and changed daily for several days. Superficial sutures are removed after 4 days and lid margin sutures 3 days later.

Plate 18-1, cont'd

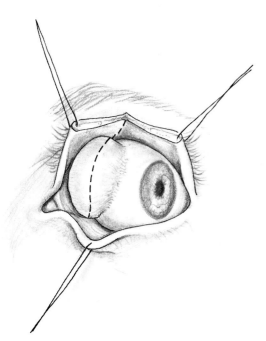

D, Following lid incision, extent of tumor is evident.

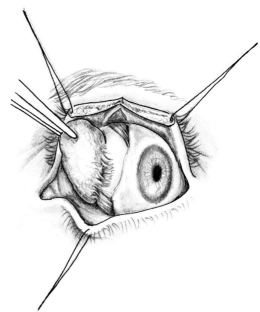

E, Excision of tumor from underlying tissue.

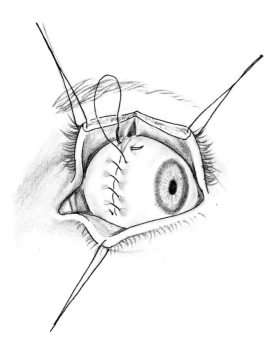

F, Conjunctival layer of incision being closed.

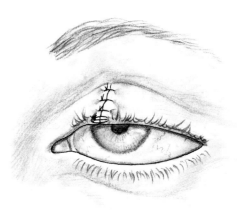

G, Transmarginal laceration closed.

The most useful procedure for exploration of the retrobulbar space is the lateral orbitotomy. This approach offers accessibility to tumors in the area between the periorbita and muscle cone (hemangiomas, for example) and within the muscle cone (optic nerve gliomas and cysts). In addition, the lateral orbitotomy is the procedure of choice for excision of tumors that are located posteriorly and anterior tumors with posterior extension.

In this procedure, performed with the patient under general anesthesia, a horizontal incision is made just temporal to the lateral canthus over the lateral orbital rim and extended to the periosteum. The incision is extended back far enough to afford a view of the entire lateral orbital wall (Plate 18-2, A). The skin and subcutaneous tissue are then undermined above and below the incision, and the wound edges are retracted, usually with a self-retaining retractor.

At this point a 6-0 silk suture is passed through the lateral rectus muscle, and the globe is rotated medially. At the periosteal level, a Bard-Parker blade is used to incise the periosteum, which is reflected from the bone (Plate 18-2, B). This incision is made parallel to the margin of the lateral orbital rim and is extended 10 mm above and below the horizontal canthal incision. A periosteal elevator is helpful in making the dissection.

Plate 18-2

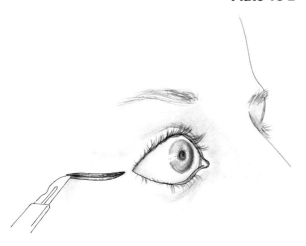

A, Lateral canthal incision made down to periosteum.

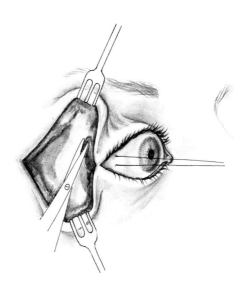

B, Periosteum incised and reflected from bone.

A bone flap about 20 mm long is then created on the lateral orbital wall and mobilized (Plate 18-2, *C* and *D*).

A Stryker saw is used to cut through the lateral orbital rim. The globe should be adequately protected at this time with a ribbon retractor or lid plate. The Stryker saw should be angled so that the superior cut is turned downward to avoid the cranial vault. The lower cut is angled slightly upward so that the saw enters the orbit and not the maxillary bone (Plate 18-2, *E*).

Plate 18-2, cont'd

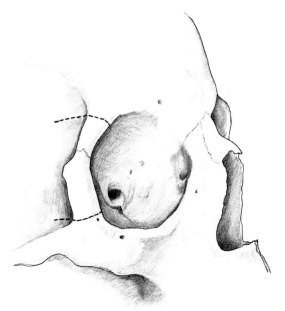

C, Bone flap to be mobilized.

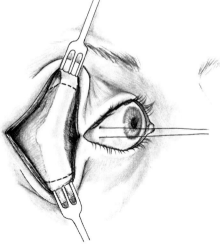

D, Suture passed through lateral rectus and extent of bone flap outlined.

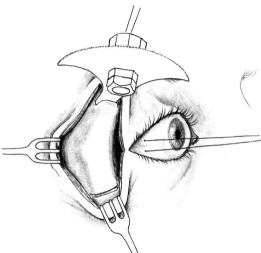

E, Stryker saw used to cut through orbital rim.

The lateral orbital rim is then grasped with a hemostat and reflected posteriorly, with the thin bone of the temporal fossa cracking easily (Plate 18-2, F). This bone flap may be removed or rotated outward. We prefer to remove the bone, because this permits some expansion of the orbital contents postoperatively, should this become necessary because of increased intraorbital pressure. This approach also gives good exposure and access to the retroorbital space. If necessary, the bony opening can be increased in size with a rongeur.

The periorbita is now visible. It is carefully cut and separated with a horizontal incision (Plate 18-2, G). The lateral rectus muscle is usually located at this time and a suture passed around it so that it can be retracted. Exploration of the orbit should be performed with the utmost care and with microscopic supervision. Even encapsulated masses should be so handled. Hemostasis should be meticulously maintained at all times.

The wound is closed with 5-0 chromic catgut suture used for the subcutaneous tissue. If the bone flap is replaced, it need not be wired. The skin is closed with 6-0 silk suture. A light dressing is applied.

Postoperatively the dressing is changed daily for several days. The silk sutures are removed after 4 to 5 days.

Plate 18-2, cont'd

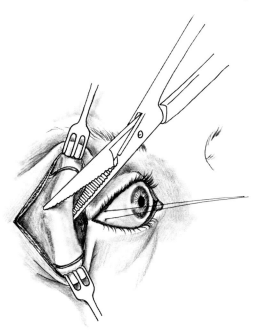

F, Bone flap mobilized with hemostat.

G, Orbital contents exposed.

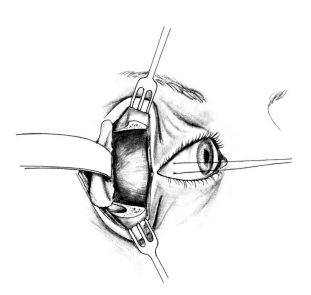

INDEX

224

X

Z